Mom's Journey

Readers' Reviews

"A quick easy read with a lot of information."

- *Mark Russell*

"Valuable personal information the medical profession does not address. With insight, experiences and resources that can assist you prior to and after the diagnosis."

- *Paul Naehring*

"Whit – I cannot properly describe how impressed I am. You did wonderfully – and I applaud you."

- *Brian O'Donnell*

"I just finished your book, and like Andrea found it impressive, powerful, and compelling. I think your book is not only a "Guy's Guide," but it will be helpful to anyone who is dealing with a parent or loved one suffering from dementia."

- *Michael Rapp*

Mom's Journey

A Guy's Guide
To Navigating A Parent's Journey
Through Dementia/Alzheimer's

By

Whitney Harrison Carnes

Cover Photo:
Pictured with draft horses; Mom, Anna Jean Harrison, 5 years old
on the family farm in Lewis County, Kentucky.
Circa 1937

Dedication

This book is dedicated to the memory of my mother and all the caregivers navigating the devastating journey that is dementia.

Also, to my sister Shelly. Without her knowledge, guidance, and support, I don't know how I would have made it through.

Table of Contents

Acknowledgements i

Foreword iii

Introduction..vi

Denial 1

Stage 1.. 5

Stage 2.. 15

Happy New Year.. 20

Seven Months Later 23

Another Move 27

The Wheels Fall Off.. 35

Take Two 44

The Jinx Is On 50

Stage 3.. 53

Afterword: Present Day 54

Time to Move.. 56

Appendices.. 61

    Montreal Cognitive Assessment Test (MOCA)................................ 63

    Takeaways 64

    Risk Factors 66

    Warning Signs 68

    Alzheimer's Myths 70

    7 Stages of Alzheimer's Symptoms 73

    The Dementias 76

    Choosing a Residential Care Facility.. 79

    Brain Apps 85

    References and Resources.. 87

Acknowledgements

I would like to acknowledge the following people for their help and support through this effort: Leslie Marsh; Jeanne Hannan; Kristen Heimerl; Chuck Hurd; Elizabeth Griesmer; Tom Martin; Kate Campbell; and Jennifer Sauers and Kristi Woodworth at Beyond the Trees Publishing.

Thank you all.

Foreword

The following story is about my mother and our struggle with dementia/ Alzheimer's disease. I say "our struggle" because this disease can be almost as devastating to the caregivers as to the patient.

There are as many stories as there are people with dementia/Alzheimer's disease. I'm sure you have heard the common questions, "Does your mom know your name? Does your dad know who you are? Did you have to take back the car keys?" From a distance, people with dementia may all seem alike. It is not until you get up close and personal that you see the variations on a theme. Every person has a different personality; therefore, this disease will affect each person in a unique way. There will be many parallels encountered in every story; but in the end, everyone's journey is different. I liken it to Harley-Davidson motorcycles, from a distance they all look and sound the same. It is not until you get up close that you can see the subtle differences.

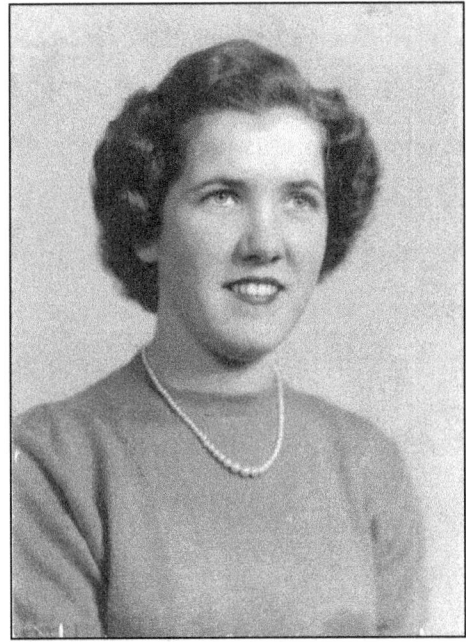

1951 - Mom's (Jean) Senior Year Photo from Lewis County High School (KY)

Mom's Journey is a guide for anyone who has a loved one going through this disease. Some of what happened in our journey may not be as relevant to what you experience. But, some situations might be spot on. This guide is geared a little more toward men. During my mother's illness, the self-help books I found were either written by women or health care professionals; and from my point of view, had too much emotional content which made me skip pages to get to the next chapter, or were hard reads with too much professional jargon. Do to that frustration; *Mom's Journey,* is a short easy read, with useful information gathered from my experience and research.

I have talked with a few men going through this with their parents in the beginning stages of dementia and found all of them angered with the situation. Not angry with the parent, but at the helplessness they feel because they don't understand what is going on. They were in denial and coming to other conclusions in an attempt to make the parent's dementia something tangible so they can understand it. I know how most males think and act. Hide the emotions, get to the point, and look for the answers so we can fix the problem. If we can't fix it we feel useless. I was guilty of this myself in the beginning. We understand heart attack, skin cancer, and diabetes because there is cause and effect with these diseases. This makes them understandable, thus real. Believe me, dementia is real but it is not understandable.

That being said, females may have a better understanding of why their father or brother isn't being as understanding and cooperative as they wish as they deal with a family member who has dementia. It helps to guide them a little and above all, be patient. In time they will adjust and accept the disease for what it is. I know I am painting this perspective using a broad brush. All men don't share the same emotional framework. Some will dive right in and help from the beginning, and some will need to test the waters before jumping in. Sadly, some men will simply disengage and watch from a distance, contributing nothing.

My hope for all who read this is to educate and prepare you for what may come your way on a physical and emotional level so you can understand and handle the journey a little easier. It wasn't until I educated myself on the subject through books and Alzheimer's literature that I overcame the anger and started to deal with the real problem at hand. We sought the best care we could for our mother, while keeping her dignity intact.

Introduction

Alzheimer's and Vascular Dementia/Vascular Cognitive Impairment (VCI), fall under the broader diagnostic category called dementia. Dementia literally means "mind away" or "deprived of mind." They are both complex, chronic, progressive diseases for which there is no definitive treatment and to date, no cure. Alzheimer's happens in stages. When we (my sister Shelly and I) were going through this with Mom in the late 1990s, the scientific community defined it in 3 stages; currently the professionals define 7 stages in which the disease progresses. With Alzheimer's, the disease progresses in a slow gradual downward curve. With VCI, the disease progresses in a downward stair-step pattern, due to mini-strokes (Transient Ischemic Attacks) inflicting the damage. Regardless of the stages, the progression is as different as the people and their personalities who experience the disease. The old adage is, "Once you have seen a person with Alzheimer's, you've only seen that person with Alzheimer's."

At present, a definitive Alzheimer's or VCI diagnosis cannot be achieved until an autopsy is performed. Even with all the imaging technology available today, brain scans usually cannot be conclusive evidence to pinpoint the actual type of dementia. Genetic testing is available to show if a person is at risk of getting Alzheimer's, but not conclusive evidence for the possibility of having mixed dementias. Blood tests are also used to rule out vitamin deficiencies like B12 or hypothyroidism or other symptoms that mimic Alzheimer's. If found, these can be treated to reverse the symptoms that were thought to be dementia. Doctors and health care workers can diagnose this disease by observing and testing the patient and questioning family members on their loved one's loss of intellectual thinking and impaired memory. After clinical examinations, around twenty to thirty percent of suspected Alzheimer's cases prove to be something other than Alzheimer's such as: Parkinson's, Huntington's, Multiple Sclerosis, Lewy Body, (to name a few) or in our case, VCI disease.

The most common test used for complaints of memory problems is the Mini Mental State Examination (MMSE). It is designed to help diagnose dementia and to assess the progression and severity. The MMSE is a series of questions that takes around twenty to thirty minutes to complete. It assesses mental abilities, including memory, attention, and language – but is not conclusive. If every question is answered correctly the maximum score is 30. In general, scores between 27 and 30 are considered normal; however, getting a lower score does not mean that a person has dementia. For example, highly educated people may find the questions too easy, while poorly educated people may find the questions too difficult. The test may also be difficult for those with learning disabilities, hearing impairments and language barriers.

Here are some sample questions:

Orientation to time: The clinician asks, "What is today's date?" "What year is it?" "Who is the President of the United States?"

Registration: The clinician states, "I'm going to say three words. You say them back to me when I stop." A few minutes later the clinician asks if the person remembers those three words. This may be repeated again.

Naming: The clinician points to a pen or pencil and asks the patient, "What is this object?"

Reading: The clinician gives the patient a sentence to read, such as "Raise your right hand." Then the patient is told, "Please read this and do what is says."

The MMSE was developed in the mid-1970s. There is another test that was designed in the 1990s that some consider a better alternative; the Montreal Cognitive Assessment test (MOCA). Like the MMSE, it takes around thirty minutes to administer but goes into greater detail. A sample of this test is in the appendix. Both tests were given to my mother. In one particular case a doctor administered them mixed together.

At present it is estimated that 5 million people in the United States are living with Alzheimer's. In 2010 there were 35.6 million people worldwide diagnosed with dementia. Two thirds lived in low to middle income countries. There is a 5 percent chance of acquiring some type of dementia over the age of 65, and a twenty to forty percent chance over the age of 85. The chances of acquiring some form of dementia increases with age; the rates are higher with women older than 65. The lifetime risk of acquiring Alzheimer's after age 65 is one out of six for women as opposed to one out of eleven for men. This is due in part by women generally living longer than men. Women over 60 are two times more likely to acquire Alzheimer's than breast cancer over the remaining years of their lives.

Usually, most people with dementia die from other preexisting conditions; however, dementia/Alzheimer's is the sixth leading cause of death in the United States claiming around 500,000 souls each year.

Dementia causes death by forgetting - forgetting how to keep the heart beating, forgetting how to keep kidneys functioning, or forgetting how to eat.

Denial

Mom was 65 when her journey began and considered to be relatively young to start showing symptoms of dementia. Since her divorce from our father (1981), Mom had problems managing money and never settled into a somewhat stable lifestyle. She was substitute teaching in Northern Kentucky plus receiving a monthly Ohio State Teachers Retirement pension, but she never seemed to have enough money to

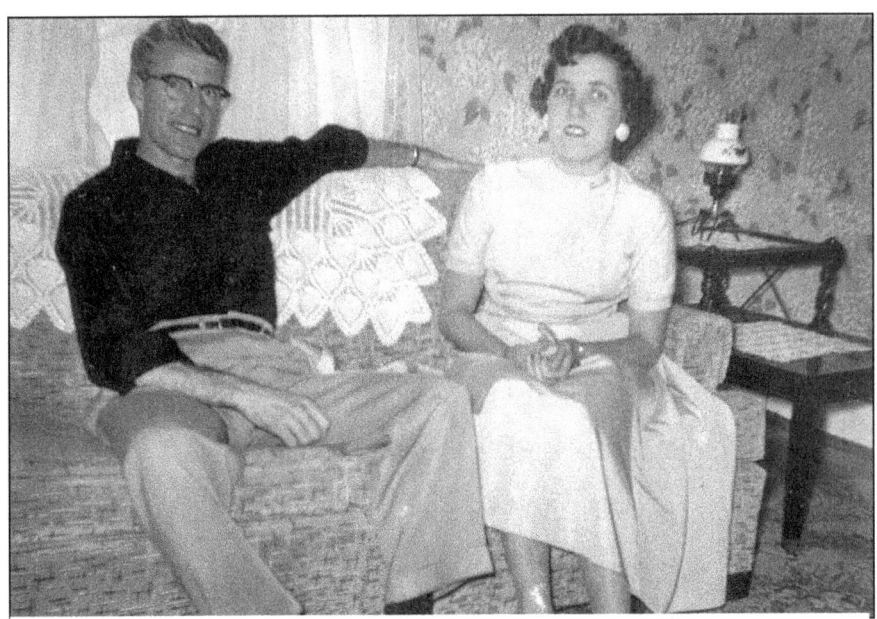

Mom and Dad (Ronnie and Jean), 1956.
They had been married one year.

make it through a month without bank penalties and late payment reminders in the mail. She spent money with little to no regard to priorities or budgets. My sister, Shelly, and I tried to help Mom with her money issues; but she would get very angry and refuse to talk about it.

This should have been the first flag that something was wrong, but as with most children experiencing this kind of behavior for the first time with a parent, we made up excuses and slipped into denial. We would justify her actions by thinking, "She's too young for Alzheimer's. That only happens to older people; she's just getting a little senile." This behavior went on for another year. One day out of the blue, I received a call from Shelly informing me that Mom put all her furniture in storage and was now living with her older sister in Columbus, Ohio. I had no clue that Mom had been thinking about moving; but after the shock of dealing with this news dissipated, Shelly and I came to the conclusion that this was probably what Mom needed all along; her sister, a role model. Our aunt was seven years older than Mom, divorced, living alone, teaching, still sharp as a tack, and seemed to enjoy Mom's company.

During this two year period, Shelly and I visited many times and found Mom to be happy and content. Then one weekend during the summer of 1999 I drove up from Cincinnati to visit. Upon arrival, Mom was crying and couldn't explain why. The whole day she was depressed and distant. When it was time to leave I asked her if she would like to come back to Cincinnati and stay with me for a while. That "while" turned into 2 years.

Mom still drove a car around well enough for not knowing the neighborhood. She acquired a part-time job shuffling pens and papers at an H & R Block a few miles away and would travel around 90 miles north to Columbus to visit her sister every other weekend. I became her Power of Attorney and canceled her checking account. I tried to review her financial situation through various canceled checks and any receipts or documents I could get my hands on. This became futile at best for lack

2

of any paper trail. I wondered how she was going through her monthly pension with nothing to show for it. I would discuss it with her, but like in the past, she would be on the defensive and get angry with me. I discovered months where her checking account accrued over $90.00 in overdraft charges. I also found out for the two years she lived in Columbus she never made a single payment for her storage unit. I was lucky enough to catch it just one month away from all her belongings going to auction. This obviously put a strain on me financially as I had to pay off the balance and move all of her belongings into my basement. Shelly also found out that Mom didn't contribute any money toward bills while living with her sister. Our aunt said that Mom spent all her money on clothes and partying. This was not the mother we knew. Her personality from a caring and giving person changed to curt and apathetic. This additional change in behavior should have been the second flag showing my sister and me that something was wrong.

As the months rolled by I started to notice her short-term memory slipping and that she had problems performing familiar tasks. For instance, we would set the table for dinner. Then, while I was out of her sight (I was actually outside grilling) Mom would sometimes put all the dishes back in the cabinet thinking, I guess, that we had already eaten. Sometimes she would push the buttons on the wireless phone while holding it toward the TV as if she was trying to change the channels. To be honest, I have also made this mistake. The difference is that through cognitive reasoning, I caught myself doing it and didn't need to call for help. There were times, usually in the evening, when she would have to think hard about how to get from one room to another. She would stand up, take a few steps, stop and look around while wringing her hands.

3

Then she would usually say something to the effect of, "Now I remember, silly me," and proceed on. There would be bad days like this and there would be good days when I almost thought nothing was wrong.

As touched on briefly in the introduction, this is the first stage of the disease that in some cases leads family members to bicker with one and other. There is usually one member in the family that is the "point person", the one who has the most contact with the loved one in question. This is the person who sees the changes in behavior and is trying to rally the troops for help. The others that don't have much contact are often the ones in denial. Since they have infrequent contact, when they call or visit it may be on the "good day." They will argue and put up defenses with the point person because they don't notice or understand the behavioral issues. They accuse the point person of exaggerating the situation: "So she didn't turn the burner off as fast as you would have liked." "So he took two wrong turns to the grocery." "So what if she put her purse in the refrigerator."

I was lucky, as Shelly was on board with me from the beginning. I have no solution to pass along to end the family bickering. What I found out though, is the bickering starts to subside and the family starts coming together after one of two things happen: either the point person gets another sibling on their side providing some needed support, or sadly, the loved one in question hurts themselves or someone else.

Stage 1

On occasion, Mom would get lost driving to and from Columbus which was a route she had driven all her adult life. She would also get lost to and from work and not realize it until she was miles away from her destination. Mom would pull into a convenience store, get the location from the clerk, and call me. I would drop what I was doing, drive to that location and have her follow me home. (I tried getting her to use a cell phone but with the small numbers and features, she couldn't negotiate it.) One day she got lost driving home from Columbus. Again, she called from a convenience store on the other side of town. I told her to stay put; and I would drive there, and she could follow me home. When I arrived a half hour later, she had already left. The convenience store clerk remembered her and told me that she asked for directions to a city in Kentucky. I drove home and called the police. I gave the police a picture of Mom so they could start the missing person's procedure on TV and radio if she had not returned by noon the next day. It was a long night of phone calls and worry. The next morning, at 10:00 a.m. she pulled in my driveway with not a care in the world and completely oblivious to the situation. Shelly and I interrogated her thoroughly and finally got the answers - and the car keys. We found out she had driven to our old neighborhood (about 25 minutes northwest of Cincinnati where we were raised and where she had taught school) and stayed all night at a motel. She could remember how to get back to our old hometown, but not to my house where she'd been living for many months now. Yet by the next morning, something must have clicked because she figured out how to drive back home.

At this point, Shelly and I realized that something was definitely wrong. Again, we saw more personality changes in relation to her disorientation to place and time, her memory loss, and how she frequently got lost while driving. It was time to seek professional help and get some answers.

As you can imagine, getting the car keys from your parent could be a real battle. We were lucky that Mom didn't put up much of a fight. When this time comes in your journey and you know that it might get ugly and emotional, I suggest having the doctor break the news. This takes some pressure off you; and you might not come off as the bad guy.

Within a 2 month period we went to 4 doctors. A geriatrics specialist diagnosed her with depression caused by possible past alcohol abuse; he thought she was too young for Alzheimer's. In less than 20 minutes, a psychiatrist diagnosed her with VCI with an element of depression, but ruled out Alzheimer's. An internal medicine doctor diagnosed Mom with Alzheimer's, but wanted to schedule an MRI to confirm his diagnosis. Holding her MRI results in hand, another physician, - a neurologist, diagnosed Mom with VCI with a component of Alzheimer's. A mixed dementia.

So now what? We had four different diagnoses from 4 doctors, all flirting with dementia. We believed the neurologist's diagnosis was more accurate due to strokes occurring frequently in our family history; plus, VCI had been the disease that took the life of her mother. The neurologist also advised us that Mom could safely stay with me unattended during the day, but it would be a good idea to start looking and preparing for housing that would be better suited for her deteriorating condition.

I'd like to point out here in regard to the geriatric doctor's diagnosis is the depression element. Depression runs hand-in-hand with dementia. Depression and bipolar disease mimic Alzheimer's and should always be considered as a possible diagnoses. The onset of depression is usually more rapid than the onset of dementia symptoms. During this time, Mom displayed the classic symptoms of depression. She experienced significant weight loss, appeared hopeless and helpless along with her declining behavioral and intellectual skills. Research indicates that in around 30 percent of dementia cases, treatable depression accompanies and exaggerates the symptoms, and, as in our case, antidepressant medications were prescribed to help alleviate the symptoms.

Shelly and I discovered that there is a lot of help for the elderly, but we really had to work hard to find it. We contacted Senior Services and they referred us to a senior center nearby. The center had a bus that came by twice a week and took Mom to the facility for activities and contact with people her age. We were lucky that Mom eagerly took to the bus transportation. I can only imagine how difficult it could have been if too much pride had gotten in the way.

I remember Mom dressed to-the-nines, and both of us standing at the front door waiting for the bus to arrive. I watched her get on the bus, introduce herself to the driver, "Hi, I'm Jean, what's your name?" She found a seat and waved to me as the bus pulled away. For an instant it was as if she were 6 years old climbing aboard the school bus for her first day of school. I closed the door and wept uncontrollably. I believe this is when the reality of the situation hit me - I was the parent now.

Mom enjoyed the Senior Center and continued her visits for around 6 months. The staff said Mom was a joy. She helped them with small duties that she could handle, and she "livened up" the place because she liked to dance with the men that were able. During this time

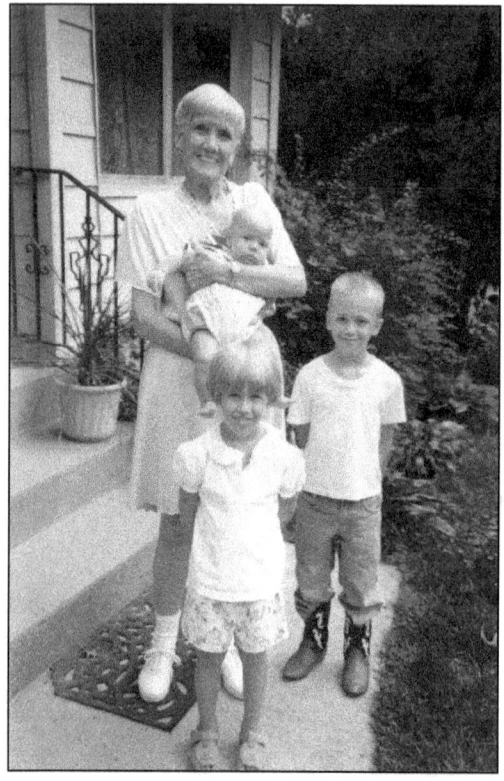

she was also on a vitamin and Alzheimer's medicine regime; and I felt comfortable leaving her alone during the day.

The next door neighbors were aware of Mom's condition and kept an eye on her when it was possible. Mom loved children so it was good to see her interact with them. Two of the older children would walk with Mom three blocks away to the drug store with only one turn to negotiate during the trip. They told me

Mom with Braden, Emily and baby Gabe before a walk to the drugstore.

that Mom knew the way there but she could not remember the way home and would forget to make the turn on the street we lived on. They would hold her hand and guide her home. (I did not know of this until a couple of years later. Apparently Mom would go next door first and ask if they wanted to go for a walk to the store. I wonder now if there was something going on in Mom's head that suggested to her that she needed the help from the children. To the best of my knowledge, she never walked to the store alone). It is very important that you make the neighbors aware of your family member's condition. Don't try to hide or be embarrassed by it. Your neighbors can be very helpful as a second set of eyes because you never know when you may have to step out for a minute or be out of sight doing laundry or cooking. That's all the time it takes for your loved one to be out the door and gone, and your neighbors can be of great help if they notice your parent walking away from home alone.

After 2 years of living with me and being alone during the day I could tell that boredom was taking its toll. She was constantly trying to find things to fill the time such as doing small loads of laundry, vacuuming every day, and ironing things that didn't even need ironing. She always turned the iron off, but sometimes never turned it on. In her mind nothing was wrong, and she would somehow justify her actions. Another time, I came home one afternoon to find Mom sitting with a strange man in the living room. I politely escorted him out and found that he was a Jehovah's Witness. He told me he'd been there for about an hour and found Mom to be engaging; but stated, he also felt something was not quite right with her.

I tried to explain to Mom that she shouldn't let strangers in the house, and that she should keep the door locked. She had an answer for everything and refused to listen to what I said. It was at this point I learned the number one lesson in dealing with people with dementia: just go along with them. Do not correct or argue or raise your voice. This will only intensify an already bad situation. You can still reason somewhat with them at this stage if you simply disengage and go along for the ride. For example, I found that if I needed Mom to do something, I made a request or positioned it as if it were her idea. Instead of saying, "It's late and you need to go to bed." I would say, "You said you had a busy day today, Mom. You must be tired – are you ready for bed?"

It was about this time we found an affordable and clean senior living community. The doctors agreed that Mom was no danger to herself and that being with people her age would be good for her. We moved her into a one-bedroom apartment (I did disconnect the stove, and for 2 years she never knew) and she took to it with ease. She had always been sociable, and she made friends fast. Although this was not assisted living, the complex was secured 24 hours with a doorman. The facility provided three meals a day in the community dining room; and there was a nurse you could hire if needed. Mom stayed stable for a while, but as we expected, the disease slowly progressed. After about 18 months she was showing more changes in behavior such as increasing disorientation and problems with abstract thinking. We noticed that Mom got progressively messy, piling clothes on the bed and sleeping on the couch with her clothes on. (I understand that sleeping on the couch while wearing clothes is common with dementia/Alzheimer's patients.) She would reminisce of her days as a schoolteacher and sometimes think that she had to teach the next day. She would walk the halls in a restless manner during late evening and night. (This behavior is common with dementia/Alzheimer's and is known as "sundowning.") She would need to be reminded to change her clothes. Mom could physically change her clothes, but she had to be talked through each step, as she had trouble with zippers and matching socks and shoes and appropriate clothing for the season. Other little problems arose too, such as remembering how to negotiate the thermostat. Many times during the winter she would turn on the air conditioning. Mom also had to be reminded to eat. Sometimes she would sit down at the table and halfway through the meal she would stand up and walk away. Usually, a staff member or resident would go to her room and bring her back to the table. She would take other people's items from the laundry room, fold them, put them neatly away and swear that they were her clothes. Sadly, the pattern of impaired thinking, loss of intellectual skills, and disorientation of time and place was getting worse.

As the doctor had told us, she would probably need to go to an assisted living facility in 2 to 3 years from the time she was diagnosed. It was time to start looking again. This would be another long and exhausting search. We are not a family of wealth, and at this time in our state of Ohio, there was no help from Medicare/Medicaid to offset assisted living expenses. Under state law only nursing homes qualify for aid. However, we found services within the county and state that will not only find money for you if you qualify, but will lead you in the right direction for assistance and answers to your questions. We talked with Senior Services, Alzheimer's Association, Lifespan, county services, and various caregivers we met along the way. We found a little help financially and a lot of caring and guidance from these outstanding services and people. The more people you bring into your circle, the more help you will receive.

We visited at least 5 nursing homes and talked with 6 assisted living facilities. The tip here is to visit them unannounced. You will really get to see what's going on instead of the staged production you receive when you make an appointment. (And I cannot stress this enough: if you walk into a facility and smell feces…turn around and walk out.) Mom wasn't ready for the nursing home environment as she could still do

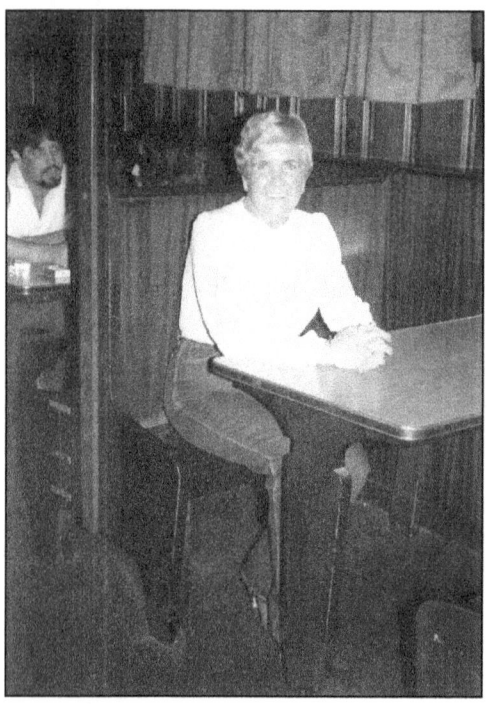

Jean when she was 50 years old, in 1982.

some things for herself. She just needed assistance and guidance on normal, daily routines. Assisted living is what we needed, but we became really discouraged at the cost. The facilities ranged from 5 to 10 thousand dollars per month. Through sheer luck we discovered a facility that would negotiate with us. They met Mom and decided that she really wouldn't need much assistance in her present condition. No walker or chair

was needed, she was not incontinent, she had no special dietary needs; we just needed caregivers to look after her daily requirements. My sister and I agreed with the facility's proposal of 50% off the monthly fees, and we soon moved Mom in. Don't be afraid to negotiate. Just like any other business, assisted living communities have quotas and financial goals, too.

Unlike her earlier move to the senior living community, Mom had a hard time adjusting to her new home. She cried and became very upset. She asked me what she did to deserve this, what was wrong with her? Was she as crazy as all the other people in here? I spent the first night with her and explained the situation. I had to repeat a lot of things and at times was positive she was understanding me. But in the end I suspect she just appreciated the company. Most of the residents were older and in bad shape; most used walkers, wheelchairs, or were bedridden. The residents who could get around on their own appeared to have some kind of dementia, and Mom picked up on that right from the beginning. Although her cognitive functioning had declined, she was still able to notice the drastic change between the friends she had left at the other facility and those who appeared in quite bad health in her new home.

It was always recommended to us that we tell Mom the truth about her diagnosis of VCI/ Alzheimer's, but Shelly and I didn't feel comfortable with using those words around her because her mother and two sisters had succumbed to this disease, and she always feared getting it herself. It completely terrified her. Our way of responding to Mom's question of, "Why am I here and, am I going crazy?" was this: "Mom, just because others living here seem to be crazy doesn't mean that you are. You are not crazy, but you do have a memory problem. Remember the mini strokes your mom had? Well you have had one or two just like your mom, and they have affected your memory. Remember we took your car keys because you kept getting lost? The doctors think you will be a lot better here with nurses and other people to help you when you need it. All you have is a little memory loss, not Alzheimer's."

We told her a half-truth; enough that she understood why she was there. She never brought it up again. It still took 3 weeks for her to feel comfortable with her new surroundings, and 3 weeks for me to stop feeling guilty. A lot of over-thinking, second guessing, and guilt can afflict the patient's loved ones.

I was fortunate to have guidance and support from my sister. I can only imagine the terror and helplessness one would feel going through this alone. My suggestion would be to surround yourself with good friends and relatives that would be eager to help. Don't be afraid to ask them to watch your loved one while you take a break for your wellbeing. Due to your loved one's condition, there will be some friends and relatives that will feel uncomfortable being around them. That's okay, they can help by being there for you – dinner, a couple of beers, a ball game. Be aware of their comfort level and don't abuse the relationship. There are plenty of in-home services available that can help with house cleaning, feeding, and nursing needs too.

Stage 2

By now her condition had deteriorated again. The doctor warned us that we could expect a drop in her condition due to the trauma of the move. Sometimes she would complain of men in her room who wouldn't leave when she wanted to change clothes. These men were TV news anchors. I did not try to reason or explain this to her, I simply turned off the TV.

In some cases television and dementia don't mix. Mom, for a while, had trouble with this. She would also ask me to lock the sliding bathroom door, as she didn't

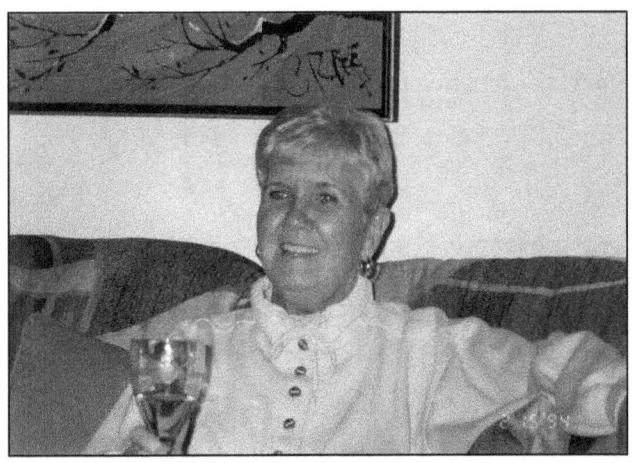

Jean at age 61.

want the kids down the street to walk into the house during the night. I broke my rule and tried to explain that this was an inside door to her bathroom not an outside door to the yard. She looked at me as if I had lobsters growing out of my head. This kind of confusion went on for about 3 months then ceased to exist.

It had now been 4 years since she was diagnosed with what we felt was the correct diagnosis, VCI with a component of Alzheimer's and we had her on mainly two Alzheimer's drugs, Reminyl®, and Namenda®. These drugs do only one thing; slow down the progression of the disease.

But I have nothing to compare what the advancement of the disease would have been like without them. They probably did some good, but in 5 years she went from having a part-time job to thinking that Peter Jennings was in her room watching her undress. Professionals say all Alzheimer's patients are impacted differently by the disease and how it advances. This being said, I am grateful that the drugs slowed the progression at any pace so that Shelly and I could spend quality time with Mom and (at least we think) that Mom was aware that we were there for her. The quicker you can get a loved one diagnosed and on medication, the better chance there is of slowing the progression of the disease and enhancing the quality of life for all involved.

It was one week away from Thanksgiving 2004. Mom had become incontinent and was wearing Depends®. She had problems with abstract thinking, and her disorientation of time and place had drastically increased. A simple car ride confused and frustrated her. Memory loss was also advancing. In regard to Mom's VCI/Alzheimer's, she displayed (like in the warning signs) short-term memory loss. She still recognized my sister and me, and she still recognized old friends of hers and relatives. What happened was that she forgot that they just visited her only minutes after they had departed. Anyone who was meaningful in her life up until 10 years before she was diagnosed, she was more likely to remember than not. However, she had already forgotten her best friend that she made at the previous facility 1 year ago, and she didn't remember any names of the staff except the head nurse which was my sister's friend from high school. She remembered Dad, but not their divorce or his death. We also noticed that her language skills had severely dropped off. She had a difficult time putting into words what she wanted or felt. We were pretty certain that this Thanksgiving would be the last one in which Mom would be able to comfortably travel from the facility to my sister's house. We also made the decision that after the first of the year we would take Mom off the Alzheimer's medications and let nature take its course. The nurses and doctor agreed that the meds weren't working anymore, and advised us that we were facing the worst stage of the disease.

Surprisingly, Mom handled Thanksgiving better than we thought. There were no problems driving to and from, and she was quite engaging and funny. When I was alone with her I got her talking about her childhood and family. Shelly made sure that Mom had plenty of bathroom breaks; and she enjoyed the dogs, cat, and the *Blues Brothers* movie on TV. It seemed as if this were one of her better days, and we hoped she could handle a Christmas trip. We did notice that she was having a hard time swallowing food and medications, and appeared to have lost some weight. We had to put food on the spoon/fork before she would eat, otherwise she would just stare at the plate. Shelly figured out that if her plate was limited to one or two food items, she would try to eat. Shelly thought that too many choices confused her, therefore frustration would set in and she would withdraw. We didn't know if this was a mental or a physical problem brought on by dementia, but we noticed another decline in her mental and physical health.

We had her weighed after the holiday and blood work done. Neither were up to par. She was to have been on a high caloric chocolate drink and a fruit drink she enjoyed, but after 3 weeks nothing had changed. We started to suspect that this facility was not providing suitable basic care, and that the staff was not trained properly to handle dementia patients. We had been concerned about this for a while, and Shelly had visited nursing homes throughout the county in preparation for our next move.

We decided not to bring Mom out to Shelly's house on Christmas. She had been declining and there was a big snowstorm that had almost everything shut down. I arrived at the facility first to find

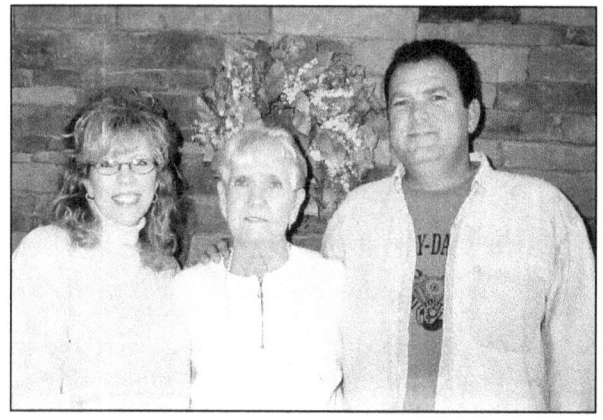

Mom at lunch alone. Most of the other residents were finished, but Mom was at the table just staring at the plate while the staff sat in the corner talking. I helped her eat her food, and when she

Mom (71 years old) with Shelly and me. The physical effects of dementia were becoming evident.

was finished I discovered that she had wet herself. As we stood up there was a foul odor and I thought she had also had a bowel movement. We walked to her room and, I put towels down so she could sit and wait for Shelly to arrive. (I could not clean my mother around that area, and doubted if I could ever get to that point if need be.) The toilet was clogged up again and her room smelled really bad. I had complained about this toilet since the first day she moved in. I knew it did not flush correctly, but the staff responded that it was my Mom's fault for stopping it up. I unclogged it and was airing out the place when Shelly arrived. She took Mom into the bathroom to change her, and discovered that not only had she urinated, but the smell was also because the staff had not bathed her nor helped her with her oral hygiene. Shelly went to the nurse's station and found out that Mom had not been bathed in two weeks.

This was the last straw. We had dealt with stopped up toilets and dried feces on the wall from an accident Mom had a month earlier. We were frustrated with employees showing up with the smell of alcohol on their breath and sleeping in the rooms of the more indigent. Over all, it reeked of sloppy care and neglect. We cleaned up Mom and the room, and had a little Christmas time with her. She was having a bad day and really didn't seem to care if it was Christmas or not.

Shelly informed me that she had picked out another facility she had heard about from the people in her Alzheimer's support group. She wanted me to take a tour and see what I thought of it, as she wanted to move Mom into it as soon as possible. I told her I would do so, and also said that I would give our 30 day notice, and she replied, "I gave it to them on the first of December."

Happy New Year

My first phone call of 2005 was my sister telling me that Mom was being rushed to the hospital. We were told that during the shower she passed out, and the nurse couldn't get a pulse. At the hospital Mom was resting and recuperating from her ordeal. After the tests were completed the doctor told us that they see too many patients from the facility that shouldn't be in emergency situations. The reason for her passing out was dehydration and anemia; as he put it, "borderline neglect." After five hours of rest and fluids she was discharged. We decided that she would live with Shelly until we could get her switched over to Medicaid and moved into the new facility Shelly had picked out. I started the process of moving Mom's belongings from her room.

The next day, as I was getting the last of Mom's belongings, the head nurse saw me and inquired of Mom's health and what the doctor's diagnosis was. As I stated what the doctor had told me, she became defensive and said she didn't believe it was the fault of either her or her staff. "Jean is in that condition," she stated, "because she just doesn't eat." I reminded her that she promised me weeks ago there would be someone with Mom at meal times to "cue" her to eat. She then said, "I've tried to sit with Jean and help her eat but she won't let me. And you know that if a person doesn't want to eat you are not going to force them." I basically left it at that and stated that I didn't feel that they were trained to handle dementia patients. The rest of the day the staff was concerned and asked about Mom. "She just won't eat," they all said. I asked about the written order that stated someone was to be with Mom to "cue" her to eat. Everyone I talked with said they didn't recall seeing anything written down regarding that instruction at all.

No one was going to take better care of Mom than my sister. I was aware of that and so was Shelly. We talked a lot about Mom's care and health, and Shelly had received a lot of feedback from her Alzheimer's support group. We were not expecting special treatment, but our minimal expectation was that she was treated with respect and dignity. Our mom was the kind of person who would put on heels and a dress to go to the grocery store because, as she said, "I am a school teacher, and you never know whom you're going to run into – maybe a

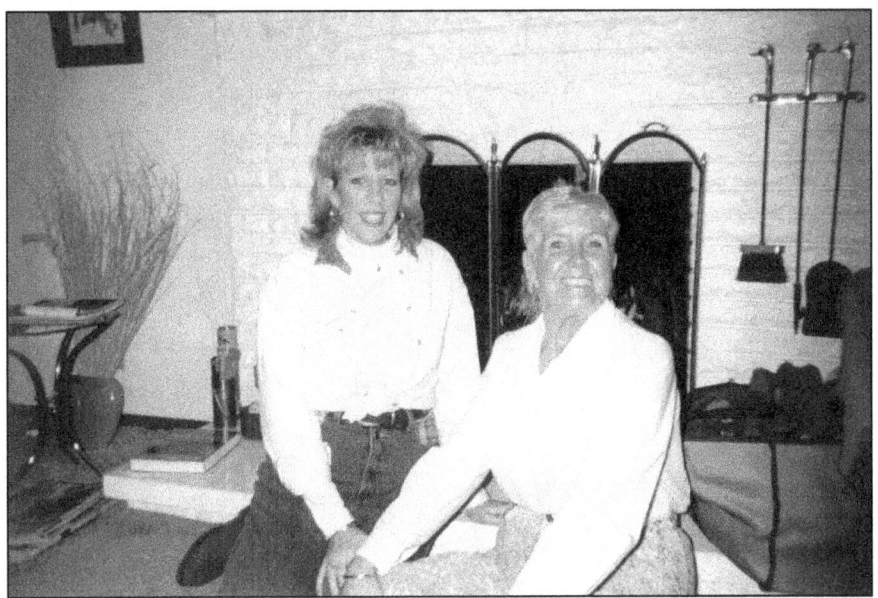

Shelly and Mom

parent or an administrator - and I want to look my best." Mom spent five days and nights with Shelly, and didn't soil herself once, and she even gained a little weight. I take my hat off to my sister. It wasn't easy. Shelly was by Mom's side 24-7. She took her to the bathroom every 3 to

4 hours, slept with her, (to make sure she didn't wander at night in strange surroundings), bathed her twice and sponge bathed her in between, cued her to eat, and constantly had her on fluids. Finally, after all the paperwork was done for the state and Medicaid, and following a visit from a doctor and social worker, Mom was able to move into the new nursing home in 5 days.

Seven Months Later

On a weekend visit Mom was teary-eyed and asked, "Who is going to love me?" Mom asked this question a lot in those days. It had been 7 months since we moved her from Boca Vista to The Gardens, a sprawling new complex with state-of-the-art facilities and room to spare. I had just left Mom as she was starting to nod off, and when I got home there was an email from my sister. I had missed a week of visiting Mom, and the day before she had cried all day because she was afraid I had been in an accident. Shelly understood that I had a hard time with the visits, but suggested that I try harder and get out there more often. I knew I should, too. Mom may not have remembered the last time I visited her, but she knew if I had or hadn't been there in a while. The two of us had a special mother-and-son bond growing up, and I felt as if I was neglecting it. I felt guilty when I was not with her, and guilty when I was. She was so afraid of not being loved.

At this facility, there were 16 people in the dementia unit stuffed away as if they were lepers. They had their own quadrant off the main floor which was away from the nurse's station. You couldn't see their area from the station because of two solid locked wooden doors obstructing the way. The other residents had piped-in music, games, activities, and parties. In the dementia unit, there was only a TV and a gospel tape playing out of little boom box that the staff herded the wheelchair-bound around to sink into a lonely and isolated abyss. We were promised that Mom would be able to participate in activities and physical therapy in the unit, but very little has actually come about. Being a new facility and needing to hire and train staff, I could give them some leeway, but I became angry and frustrated when I continued to see events and parties on the other side, yet they didn't invite the dementia patients who were well enough to participate. When we questioned the administrator about the lack of activities in the dementia area, he blamed it on budget cuts and lack of staff to safely accompany patients to events. But he did tell us that if we were present while events were going on, we could bring our mom to them (but only Mom, and not another person even if we knew the family, and if there were 2 of us assisting them due to potential lawsuits.) This aside, the place was clean and safe. The doctor changed Mom's anti-depression medicine to one with an appetite stimulator and she gained 10 pounds. She seemed now to enjoy eating and didn't need to be cued as much. The problem at mealtime was that the aides seated the patients that could walk first - sometimes 20 minutes before food was served. Almost all of them would get up and walk out and never eat their meals. We suggested that they seat the people in wheelchairs and walkers first, and then get the ones that can walk, but our comment fell on deaf ears. It seemed that a lot of logical suggestions never got attention.

Mom was still physically healthy and could get around by herself. So if she wasn't pacing the halls, she was in her room or visiting another resident, Helen. Helen and Mom got along well together and enjoyed each other's company. Although they didn't know each other's names or talk much, there seemed to be a spiritual bond they both found soothing and comfortable.

This facility was better than where she had been the previous year, but they were understaffed and, again, apathy was prevalent with a lot of the staff. For example, Mom was mobile and walked around, so we suggested that she (and the head nurse agreed) wore fresh Depends when she was put to bed, and helped into a fresh one in the morning. The aides had to change her clothes anyway, so we felt this was a reasonable request to make. For the residents who were wheelchair bound, they were put to bed naked from the waist down on a big disposable bed pad they called a chuck. That was understandable because these people couldn't get themselves out of bed and use the toilet. However, Mom could use the bathroom, and we wanted to encourage her independence in this area. We also didn't want her walking the halls naked. Plus, Mom frequently got urinary tract infections called UTIs (2 in 7 months), so we were trying to encourage the staff to pay more attention to this by keeping her dry as possible. Unfortunately, on the weekend shifts, we would often find her pajamas drenched with urine on the floor. At night the aides were putting her in pajamas without the Depends.

Shelly continually brought to my attention that they were not changing or even checking Mom. She acquired another UTI and her skin became red and split open at the pelvis. Four aides that were actually responsible and caring were let go or quit. We discussed our concerns with our social worker, and found out her sister lived in the same facility. She informed me that residents were lucky to get attended to every 6 hours because they were severely understaffed. The social worker also advised us that the facility was frequently using temporary help in the memory impaired unit. Even more distressingly, the facility was under investigation by the state. Those vulnerable and dependent people were not getting even the most basic care required under state laws. I called and emailed the administrator; but like always, he passed the blame on their budget cuts and even suggested that we were asking for too much. He also proposed that we should look for another facility if we felt that they were not providing adequate care for our mother. Our suspicion was that the new head nurse and administrator were in over their heads. This was the consensus with all of us that had family there, not just my sister and me.

Another Move

It was now October 2005. Mom had been at Rolling Hills for 3 weeks. The move from The Gardens to this facility was swift, and Mom handled it pretty well. She had good and bad days just as before. Sometimes she would cry, "This place is so beautiful, how am I going to afford it?" Unlike the last facility, this residence was staffed properly and maintained a great reputation within a small college community. They had students/interns there majoring in Geriatric Care, Psychology, and other courses of study that gave the place a high energy level not present at the other facilities. The nurse's station was adjacent to the memory impaired floor. The rooms were private and carpeted (the last place had tile floors and two residents per room). The level of cleanliness and care was evident since the facility was carpeted and smelled fresh even though there were patients who were incontinent. The staff made sure the patients went to bed wearing Depends and pajamas. They allowed residents to awaken when they wanted to, not at some morning cattle call which was convenient for the staff. We felt really good about this place, as we did the last two. Shelly was really excited but I was still reserved, and not getting my hopes up until Mom had been there for a while. The ironic aspect to this find was that Shelly discovered it while going through the Yellow Pages, and it was only 15 minutes from her home.

They had a lot of activities here. One day, they took Mom and a few others to an elementary school where they read to some children. The activities director was amazed at Mom's performance. She said that

Mom teared up as they walked into the school then pulled it together and became a teacher again. I hope that Mom felt her pride come back, even if it was for a short while. One week later they took a group to Pizza Hut® and a women's college basketball game. Activities and stimulation were a welcome upgrade from the other places she had lived.

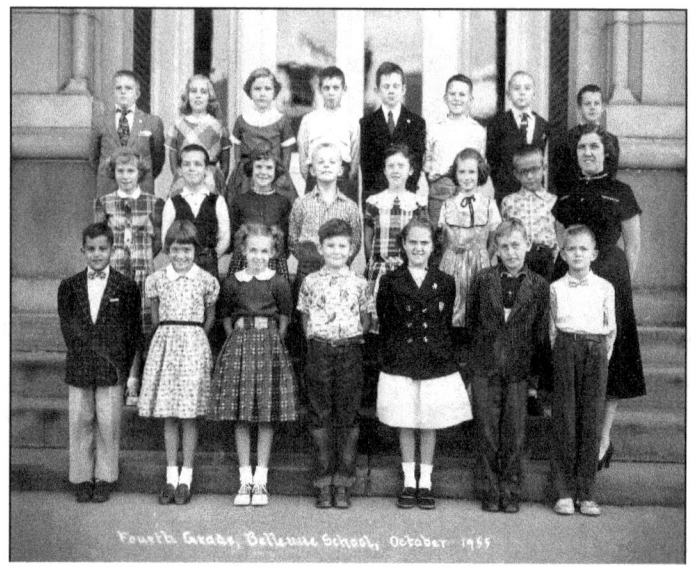

Jean was a schoolteacher. Here she was in 1955 with her 4th Grade Class at Bellevue School in Kentucky.

During one of my evening visits, I found Mom at the dining table finishing a cheesecake dessert. I talked with the nurse on duty and she informed me that Mom was slowly warming up to her new surroundings, but not wanting to take all of her meds and sometimes not wanting to get dressed in the mornings. They didn't force pills nor try to make her change clothes, as they wanted to gain her trust. As I sat beside Mom, she was happy to see me; and when I ask her how she was doing she said, "Crying but I don't know why," and started to tear up. I hugged her and suggested that we go to her house and watch some funny TV. I sat her down with the rest of her dessert and she ate it promptly with no problems. (A year before she could hardly eat by herself. I felt the improvement was due to the appetite stimulant coupled with better care and stimulating activities.) Suddenly she looked at me and said, "I have to go to the bathroom." She stood up and grabbed herself. A little too late, but had presence of mind to at least know what the urge was and what to do next. A week before, in fact, she went to the bathroom on her own with no problems. It was a quiet visit as she was not very talkative and I could not get much out of her. She said she was in some deep thought but couldn't explain it to me. She could, however, remember some words and sang along to the old songs on the *Lawrence Welk Show*.

A year ago, Shelly and I, through the advice of a doctor and nurse, were going to take Mom off the Alzheimer's medications, as they believed they were not working any more. We didn't. (Even though we did agree with their opinion at the time, we felt - in our hearts - that it would have been too cruel.) We firmly believed that the lack of attention and stimulation really pronounces and speeds up the disease. Medications and stimulation need to work together. You cannot expect optimal results without the two working hand-in-hand. There would be a time when the meds wouldn't work anymore, but that time was not now.

Mom still recognized us and remembered our childhood; yet she thought that her mother who was laid to rest in 1976 was still alive. She still knew my sister's husband of only 9 years but started to forget names of old friends and some family members in pictures around her room. This is what astonished us. Shelly married Tom soon before Mom was diagnosed, but Tom really stuck in her head. On the other hand, she was having a hard time remembering some of the teachers she had as friends and taught with for years.

It was 4 days before Thanksgiving, 2005 - Mom's birthday. She was 73. We had a little dinner at Shelly's house. Mom didn't seem comfortable. She was slowly adjusting to the new surroundings and faces of the aides and nurses at the Hills; but now at her daughter's house she seemed lost and despondent. Mom barely spoke and we had to constantly put food on her fork and cue her to eat. This was familiar territory to us and may have been in part an effect of her anti-depressant medication being changed. She was having a harder time adjusting to the new place, and the nurse took her off of the medication with an appetite booster and changed it back to Zoloft®. Mom had trouble maneuvering around the two dogs and cat at Shelly's house; and if she was not physically taken to a chair to sit, she would just stand and look helpless. Mom began to look and act very frail. She took my arm as we were leaving and almost fell twice on steps and in the yard walking to the car.

Thanksgiving found me at a fast food joint eating in my truck. Shelly and Tom stayed home. We were all depressed by Mom's condition and just wanted get through the day with as little effort as possible. Since the birthday visit, we decided it would be best for Mom not to travel anymore. Shelly and Tom saw her at lunch and helped feed her; I showed up shortly after that to find Mom in the chair dozing off. She looked great. It was her shower day and they had styled her hair. Mom was talkative with me but was making no sense whatsoever. She was going on about a little boy at school with a lisp that wanted to stay with her. She was getting ready to walk to the bus stop to see if he was all right. She continued about how he didn't have a father to love him and that all little boys need a father. She teared up as she looked at me and apologized for me not having a father. I simply said that I did and I was old enough to be a father. I directed her attention to a *Gunsmoke* TV rerun, and for a while we were back on track. Then within less than 5 minutes, she returned to the little boy story again. I got up and walked out the door saying that I was going down to the bus stop to check on him. She agreed, and that was it. (Remember, go along with the story. Trying to correct or reason with her would have been futile.) I sat her in the big chair and put her feet up as she was starting to get tired. I gave her a kiss on the cheek and said, "I love you." I had recently grown a short goatee, and she playfully recoiled and asked when I would shave that thing off. She hated it. I thought I would keep it, as it seemed to get her going. Maybe it would help with her memory of me down the road.

It had been 6 years since the diagnosis of VCI with a component of Alzheimer's. She still had these little periods of lucid thought that would come and go. I wondered if there were any cognitive thoughts in regard to her condition. Mom could be difficult at times with the staff. She didn't like to be told what to do and would talk back to the nurses and aides. She did not like loud talking or sudden movements toward her. I believe this to be common with dementia patients as they need a lot of adjustment time to acquire trust and familiarity. Sunday I found Mom in her pajamas at 2:00 P.M. The aides said that they just couldn't get her to change and since it was a Sunday they weren't too concerned. My feeling was that it wasn't that big of a deal either, but all the other patients had clothes on and we didn't want our mother looking out of place. If she knew she was walking around like that, she would be embarrassed.

That's the hell with this disease. The people with the disease don't know or care, but we do. I got her to change into her clothes for me just by saying, "Mom, it's two o-clock in the afternoon. Don't you think it's time to get out of your pajamas?" Again, if you want them to do something for you, try this simple technique. In a calm voice, position your request as a question. The aides had her changed in a matter of minutes.

Overall we were pleased with the care here, but problems started to appear. For instance, not wearing her dentures at lunch. I wondered how did she eat breakfast for that matter, and how would she be able to eat lunch. Shelly noticed that on days she was helped with her shower, Mom had bruising on her arms. Since this had been going on for a while, Shelly took pictures and showed them to the head nurse. She agreed with Shelly that they were a result of the aides holding her arms down while showering. We agreed that Mom would only be given tub baths, not showers, due to the fact that she was terrified of the shower. (Growing up, Mom never showered, she always bathed. We also thought that Mom might have mistakenly believed it was raining, and threw her arms up as if to keep her head dry.) We were disappointed to find that the two aides in question retaliated. They neglected to change her in the morning and allowed Mom to sleep in wet Depends all night and all day until their shift change. Then they wiped Mom with her pajamas and left them urine drenched on the floor! We attended the family care meeting and discussed this along with the teeth issue with the administrator; unlike the last place, the two aides were reprimanded and removed from the memory-impaired nursing unit.

During the family planning meeting (where anyone with family members was welcomed and encouraged to attend), we all brought up the problem with meals. The facility didn't have enough help at mealtime, and many of the residents were not eating. Shelly visited every Monday through Saturday at lunchtime to feed Mom. I went on Sundays. One week after the meeting, we noticed that the staff was trying to address the problem, and it seemed to be getting better.

As we noticed this improvement, Shelly began visiting every other day and became less stressed. I continued my Sunday visits and found things usually very good. Mom gained weight and seemed content. There were going to be accidents and bad days; we had to expect that and deal with it. This facility was by far the best, but we still had to address intermittent problems with care as they arose.

During one of my Sunday visits, Mom was sitting with an aide at the nurse's station dressed to-the-nines, eating Doritos®, drinking punch, and having a ball. Mom seemed not to care that I was there at all; it was good to see her this way. The aide introduced herself and said that Mom was her fourth grade teacher and one of her favorites. She intended to take exceptional care of her. Shelly and I loved hearing that; it was almost like having an extended family member watching over her at night. But after 2 weeks we found out that the administration moved her to the other side of the building where they were understaffed. These staffing changes occur often and are very frustrating to family members. It is hard enough to find the aides that want to work with the memory impaired; and when a good one arrives, it seems they always ship them off somewhere else.

Three moves in one year – no wonder it took Mom around 5 months to adapt to the new faces and surroundings. On Mother's Day, they had a tea social with a gentleman playing old piano songs. The attendance was sparse, but the residents and family who attended seemed to enjoy it. Mom sang a little with the songs that sparked her memory, but for the most part seemed not to care one way or another. Before we walked to the commons for the social, Shelly had Mom looking great by giving her a new necklace and perm. Then, Shelly took out a tube of lipstick. Mom snatched it from her hand and applied it herself. Perfectly, I might add; she still remembered how to do that!

The Wheels Fall Off

Since Mother's Day, we had 4 weeks of urine drenched pajamas and clothing. Shelly complained to the administrator and the assistant head nurse, but nothing changed. There were times you could actually wring out urine from her clothing. Again, in retaliation for our complaining, two aides left urine and feces-covered clothing in a ball on the bathroom floor or draped them over a towel bar. It was the over-night shift that were not properly checking and changing her; they allowed our mother to lie in her urine and feces all night long, and then cleaned her up before first shift arrived.

Toward the end of June, Shelly called me and said that she thought Mom had a stroke. Mom was now walking very erect with her spine arched back. Her steps were very small and unsteady. Her demeanor was distant and not very responsive; she wore an empty glossy look in her eyes. Then 2 days after this observance she passed out in the bathroom (ironically, while in the company of two aides that were assisting) and hit her head on the toilet. Shelly rode with Mom in the ambulance to the hospital. The MRI showed no new evidence of a stroke, and thankfully just a small contusion from the fall. But we were shocked to be told that the doctors had diagnosed her with a severe UTI. Her lab report revealed that the infection was almost at a toxic level and if not treated, it would have spread to other organs, and her death would have been imminent. Shelly told the attending physician the conditions Mom was subjected to, laying in urine overnight for weeks at a time. The physician, keeping in mind Mom's track record for getting UTIs, confirmed our suspicion that the lack of care was mainly to blame for the fall and her deteriorated condition.

It just so happened that a family care meeting was scheduled soon after this incident. Needless to say, Shelly and I voiced our concerns and other family caregivers chimed in with the same worries. The staff member facilitating the group said that the meetings were not designed for this type of display and attack. The 6 of us then asked, then what are we supposed to do if for 4 weeks we complained to the nurses on duty, the assistant nurse, head nurse, facility social services worker, and the administrator with no remediation? The administrator jumped out of his chair exclaiming that we were all making him look bad in front of his nurses and the facility doctor. Although the meeting became contentious, at least it was comforting to realize that we were not the only ones experiencing this problem. Shelly and I had started to get paranoid in thinking that we were asking for too much, or were we the only ones with this problem, or wondering if the aides retaliated because they heard of our displeasure with Mom's care.

Every person in the memory-impaired unit had special needs and problems, whether it was diabetes, or they were confined to a wheelchair, had dietary issues, used catheters, etc. Mom had only one concern: UTIs. She walked and could eat independently now with just a little help from the aides. She just needed to be checked and toileted periodically to help prevent infection. Mom's primary doctor had prescribed numerous medications to cure and prevent UTIs but stated that with her history and the deteriorating condition caused by her dementia she would never be completely free of UTIs. Most likely, said the doctor, it would be the cause of her death.

The first week in July rolled around, and Shelly was completely stressed out from the last few weeks and the confrontation during the meeting. She asked and I agreed to take over her duties for the entire month. I now visited on Sundays, Tuesdays, and Fridays; and kept up with Mom's laundry. The facility was an hour's drive each way, but it was really important to both Shelly and me that we work together and be there for each other. I also made an arrangement with the head nurse that we would only come to her with problems and concerns. I felt by addressing one person rather than the four nurses that work the memory impaired unit, there would be better communication, bringing better results.

Three weeks after that meeting there was noticeable improvement. I did not notice any urine drenched clothing, and Mom was more responsive and alert. It was obvious that second and third shifts had become more attentive to Mom's needs. When I visited her, I found her in good spirits; and to my relief, she was clean and dry. She was even eating better on her own. I contacted the head nurse and praised her and the staff for their efforts. I strongly believed that if you complain you'd better praise.

It was our experience that the ebb and flow of care will always fluctuate from satisfactory to borderline neglect. There is a lot of turnover in this industry, thus, the ball gets dropped from time to time. We found that about every 4 to 5 weeks we had to raise our concerns to the nurses that Mom was not getting toileted properly; or we were finding urine drenched pajamas. They always addressed our concerns, and the care generally improved for about 4 or 5 weeks. I learned to accept this as the normal procedure; however, Shelly thought differently.

Shelly was present at the facility more than I was, and she experienced more of the problems. I later discovered that she had shielded me from some issues as well.

I got a call in mid-August from Rolling Hills that they were rushing Mom to the hospital and Shelly was with her. I arrived to find Shelly with Mom in the emergency room. Mom was resting quietly and in stable condition. Shelly told me she was helping Mom to her chair after dinner and noticed Mom's arms start to tremble, her eyes became fixed and open, her breathing stopped and her face tuned an ash-like color. Mom collapsed, and they both melted to the floor. Shelly yelled, "Mom!" repeatedly, and then held her close and whispered that she loved her. After around 30 seconds, Mom blinked and whispered back, "I love you, too." Mom stayed in the hospital for 3 days. I did the day watch and Shelly stayed at night. The reason for the constant vigil was to keep Mom calm and assure her with a familiar face. After a battery of tests, it was discovered that mom had another mini stroke.

Mom was in bed for 3 days straight. After the news of a stroke, we were curious to see what had been affected. She was actually talking better, completing her sentences, and telling us some of her thoughts. It seemed that her health had actually improved! Shelly and I held Mom between us and moved her to a chair thinking that the stroke may have affected her balance through some type of paralysis. Mom was talking away and then lifted herself out of the chair and walked better than before the stroke! We checked her out of the hospital and drove her back to Rolling Hills; to everyone's surprise it was as if her condition improved to how she had been a year and a half earlier.

Shelly believed Mom's apparent recovery was divine intervention; I wanted medical knowledge and thought her doctor would be excited and want to make a case study with her. But I was told that apparently this phenomenon happens from time to time. The doctor explained to me that the place where Mom had her stroke was in an area of the brain that usually experiences little to no damage. As far as the stroke improving her condition the doctor stated, "The brain is a very complicated place. We don't know half of what really happens there. The stroke probably tripped some electrical processes that were dormant before."

We were still pleased with the positive change in Mom's condition. She could once again let us know when she needed to use the bathroom. She could recite this rhyme and inject humor into it: "The bee stung the bull on the butt and started the bull to buck. The same damn bee stung Adam and Eve and started the whole world to…" At that point in the rhyme she stops, smiles and says, "I don't say the last word."

However, she was once again confusing TV with reality. She referred to the events on TV as, "over there." She loved *Emeril* and the *Food Network*, *Gunsmoke*, and *Leave it to Beaver*. She also recapped some of what happened to her during her stroke experience. She recalled where Shelly and Tom were in the room and repeated what Shelly had said to her. Sadly but not unexpectedly, after 2 months Mom slowly slipped back to the cognitive condition she was in prior to the mini stroke.

It was now October 2006; one year at Rolling Hills and things were going fairly smoothly. We still saw the soiled pajamas from time to time and had to complain, but overall, I was happy with her care.

Shelly was concerned about Mom's weight. Mom was 125 pounds when we moved her there and now she was 144. The extra weight made it harder for her to get out of chairs and walk. She had fallen once but was not hurt. I noticed that she had problems with depth perception and patterns on the floor. She would walk normally on a solid color floor, but during a transition from solid blue to various colors with patterns, she looked down, slowed up and took shorter more careful steps. Mom's weight gain didn't bother me but it was concerning for Shelly. I believed that if Mom wanted cookies and cake and sweets, let her have them. My God, what else was there for her to look forward too! If they made her happy for that instant, so be it. Shelly, on the other hand, was concerned about the health issues. Such as when the kitchen didn't prepare the low fat meals correctly, or when the aides gave Mom junk food rather than fruit. I didn't care, as long as Mom ate and was happy.

This difference in opinion obviously divided us. The two of us were at Rolling Hills for at least 6 of Mom's meals each a week. When I was there, Mom had no problem eating on her own, and I let her take as long as she wanted. We always ate in her room rather than the dining room, as there were no distractions. I seldom gave her dessert unless it was fruit. Obviously if she was up to 144 pounds she was not starving. I did agree with Shelly though, that 144 was the top end of her desired weight. The nurses and aides told me that they do try from time to time to give Mom fruit rather than cakes and cookies, but Mom still knew the difference and desired what the rest of the group was eating. Honestly, how can you not cave in and give her a cookie or some pie?

I told Shelly that if you look hard enough at anything you will find something wrong. I believed Shelly needed to lighten up a bit, or as I told her, "You're going to stroke out." Shelly was seriously considering moving Mom in with her and Tom, two dogs, a cat, and a bird. I twice talked her out of it and hoped that this was the end of this idea. She had to get over her guilt and live her life; Mom was getting good care and was safe. In one of Mom's lucid moments, Shelly told me, she asked Mom if she wanted to move in with her and Tom. Mom looked into Shelly's eyes and said, "I would like to, but that wouldn't be fair to you and Tom. You two have your lives to lead." Out of nowhere, came a coherent thought and reply. What a crazy disease this was.

If you have read this far, you might be wondering with all these issues, why we had Mom in these facilities rather than living with one of us with the assistance of in-home-care? Fair question; I will try to answer. During this time period, the in-home-care was in its infancy, and not as prevalent as it is now. Money was also a big factor along with both Shelly and me working full time plus Shelly taking night classes to become a nurse. Believe me, there are just as many neglect and abuse stories in the in-home-care industry, too. Theft is a big problem, not only in terms of personal property but prescription medications, too. In some remote situations where the patient is bedridden and can't communicate, there have been reports of caregivers partying and using the elder's property as a front for drug activity. There have also been unfortunate accounts of overall neglect and inattention to personal hygiene and nutritional needs. No matter which avenue you chose in regard to caring for your loved one, it is very important that family members keep a watchful eye on the situation.

To my surprise, Mom was fine at Shelly's house during Thanksgiving 2006. She mostly sat in the chair next to the fire, quiet but content. She ate well and on her own. Even the car ride to and from Rolling Hills went off without a hitch. We were very pleased to get her out of the facility and to a real home with family. It is even more meaningful around the holidays, because you always wonder if this will be the last time.

Mom had fallen twice since the stroke but had not hurt herself. We believed that she was still having mini-strokes. I noticed that she was cognitively slipping again, and not as sharp as when we brought her back from the hospital. For instance, she would give no warnings for bowel movements and was not finishing sentences. She started walking a bit slower and was a little unstable (this could be the weight gain too.) She had problems with balance and the staff had found her on the floor in the bathroom and in other people's rooms. We put a pad on her chair that cued her to sit down when she attempted to stand up. If she continued, an alarm went off which let the staff know she was up and to keep an eye on her. We found that in most cases, she was either in her room with the TV on, or in the gathering room on the couch. Nevertheless, she still had a sense of humor and loved to cut up and laugh with the staff and strangers and even at my funny faces and silly jokes.

Another area that Shelly and I disagreed was letting her walk the floors picking at things on the floor and walls as if she were cleaning up. Mom believed the whole area was her home and the other people there were just visiting her. I could only imagine how frustrating it must have been for her not to be able to get around. Mom was a walker, a wiggleworm. Shelly didn't want her to fall and break a hip or become bedridden in the event she tripped and fell. I understood her side too, so I let it go. I always caved in. I realized Shelly spent more time at Rolling Hills and was also a bit overprotective. The compromise between us was that we walked with Mom every visit and requested that a staff member from the activities department walk with her daily. Mom didn't qualify for therapy because she could walk unassisted for some amount of pre-determined steps. Therapy was only prescribed for those that would show some type of improvement after or during therapy.

Take Two

Still, after all that time, out of the blue would come a cloak of guilt that lay heavy on my shoulders. It usually happened when I was with friends at the local watering hole or just out trying to have some fun. I would get a heavy heart and my eyes would well up as I thought of Mom. What was she doing? Was she happy? Was she warm and dry? Was she lonely or in pain? Had anyone said hello to her or given her the time of day? Had Shelly visited recently? I thought to myself, here I was out having fun and Mom was there, alone. God, I must be the bad son. Even when I visited I felt depressed when I left. Was it a quality visit? Did I stay long enough? Did Mom enjoy it? Did she even know I was there?

I began to hate it when my friends asked how she was doing. I knew they were genuinely concerned, and I was grateful that they were; but I was exhausted with the whole situation and would rather talk about something else. They meant well, but if I heard one more time, "Does she still know who you are?" I was afraid I was going to snap and say something I'd regret later. If only people knew that there was much more to this disease than forgetting your face and name.

I recall it was even worse when the phone rang and the caller ID showed my sister's number. I sometimes didn't want to pick it up. I knew it was going to be a problem, or a situation that needed to be addressed, seldom did we talk without Mom being the axis of the conversation. The only other phone number that rated up there in the "oh no" category was the number of the facility. It rang one morning; it was the nurse.

"Whitney, your mom has fallen and it appears that it is a stroke again. Shelly is with her and is very upset. She asked me to call you and tell you that we are taking her to the hospital." When I arrived at the emergency room, Mom was awake, dreary but otherwise cognizant and in good spirits. Shelly was by her side just like the last incident occurred.

Shelly told me that she was walking Mom from the bathroom to her chair when Mom stopped; her eyes fixed and became glassy, her mouth opened and went slack, her skin became grayish in color, her chin dropped to her chest and then her knees buckled. Shelly grabbed her, and the two of them sunk gently to the floor. Shelly yelled for the nurses while whispering in Mom's ear that she loved her. Mom had no heartbeat for two minutes. Just like the last time, Mom opened her eyes, looked at Shelly, and whispered, "I love you, too." Her blood pressure rose to 170/140, so they called 911.

Blood work, urinalysis, and a scan showed no conclusive evidence of a stroke; however, they did find that she had another severe UTI. The doctor said in older women this can really shake things up and can cause episodes like the one she had just experienced; but not to rule out another mini-stroke. Mom was released, and we had her back in time for dinner. This was the second time that Shelly had gone through this ordeal and it was obviously discomforting to her, not only in terms of the odds of it happening both times when they were together, but the spiritual ramifications it conjured up in her mind, too.

As I was feeding Mom, Shelly was in conference with the nurse on duty. So much for the agreement I had made with head nurse months ago. Again, I thought everything had been going along just fine. I soon found out that Shelly had once again tried to protect me from the problems by handling the issues herself – putting it all on her back. Apparently Shelly had become aware that a lot of Mom's pants had been soaked with urine. This led my sister to the conclusion that they were not changing Mom, and she was lying in urine soaked Depends for too long. She suspected that it was the night shift that was not toileting her because when Shelly left the facility during the day shift, she knew Mom's pants were dry. When Shelly would visit the next day, she found the pants in the hamper were wet, but Mom's pajamas were dry. Therefore it appeared that second shift was dropping the ball. Shelly had reported to the nursing staff that Mom's vagina was red and obviously the UTI was back again. I knew that Shelly had problems with 2 night shift aides, and I believed this was clouding her judgment. After Shelly left, one of the aides came to me and said that there was no way that they didn't want to take care of Mom. "We know Shelly has issues with us," they said, "but we really try hard to toilet her and check her. We love your Mom but we feel that Shelly just wants to blame us." I simply stated, "Shelly is a bit over-protective. She's not out to get anyone fired, it's just that this is our third facility, and this repeated situation just gets old after a while. We want our Mom to be clean, fed, and comfortable, just like you would want yours." I tried to be the "good cop" and assure them that I was happy with their efforts and that I would talk to Shelly. I hate conflict, but I do believe that the aides in question were not entirely at fault. As one aide said, "We know she's incontinent. Lots of times we will sit her on the toilet; sometimes she goes, sometimes she doesn't. So what's to say she would urinate five minutes later, but we wouldn't catch it until we checked her 2 hours later?"

This was a battle since day one. I could understand both sides and wanted to be on the side of my sister, but I still could not honestly blame it on one shift. Even while Mom was visiting with us during Thanksgiving, Shelly must have taken her to the bathroom every hour and still Mom urinated while sitting in the chair at the kitchen table. I did not tell Shelly of the conversation I had with the aides; I doubt I ever will.

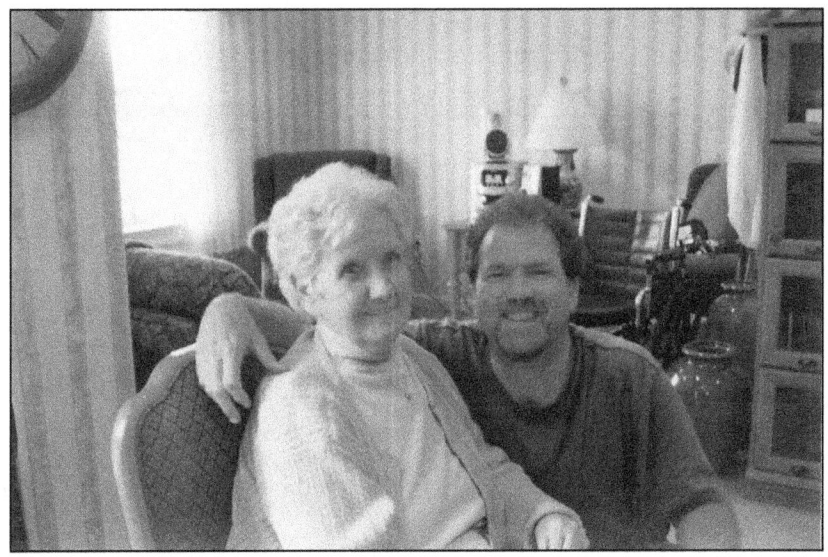

Mom and me, 2008. My favorite picture.

It was now mid-summer 2007, and I was reluctant to write anything down in my journal. Since my last entry, everything had been going great and I didn't want to jinx it. They moved all the memory impaired patients into a new Memory Support Unit, and it exceeded my expectations. They hired a new, mature experienced lady to assist with activities; and they do a lot of them, even picnics! There was always a complete staff with little turnover. This bred familiarity and brought a sense of calm and trust with the patients. First and foremost, Mom was getting changed fairly regularly and her UTIs were kept in check. Francie, one of the nurses, was really in tune with Mom. She could tell, as we could, when one was coming on by Mom's personality changes. If Mom became quiet, lethargic, and tired, she needed to be checked for a UTI.

The only problem we encountered was getting Mom's teeth brushed. Mom needed to have two cavities filled but the last two times the dentist refused to fill them because her gums were too swollen and red. I noticed that all the patients in the unit seemed to be lacking dental hygiene. In Mom's case, she didn't want to cooperate, because she had no clue what was going on. Trying to get her to open her mouth was nearly impossible, but for some reason, I was about the only one she would let brush her teeth without getting her upset.

Shelly was happy with the care Mom was receiving and took a full time job caring for indigent elderly people in their homes. I believed this was a positive step for her as she cut back her days visiting; but again, a Catch-22. Shelly's stress level was down and her guilt level was up. She continued Mom's laundry and beauty parlor visits every Friday. As for me, I visited twice a week and escorted Mom to functions that conflicted with Shelly's schedule.

As far as Mom's overall condition, not much had changed. She was a little weaker and still required a wheel chair for long walks. Going from her room to the big room (about 80 feet) she could walk with assistance, and the staff was good about walking with her to help maintain her muscle tone for as long as possible. Mom loved to watch TV with me and would laugh at the appropriate times. She still had a great sense of humor but couldn't articulate what or why something was funny. One day I got a little too focused on the TV. Mom, feeling I was ignoring her, yelled out, "Hey," and slapped my arm. I got that old "Mom" look that I thought had long gone away. Another time we were watching *Larry the Cable Guy*, and Mom laughed at the off-color humor. (Mom still thought that the people are in the TV, not on the TV) and said, "He's has to be a friend of yours, he's crazy." This was about as long a thought pattern she could express. Although few and far between, I loved them, especially when they were funny.

The Jinx Is On

No kidding. In less than 24 hours after writing that sentence about the jinx, I got a call from my sister because they were taking Mom to the emergency room. She had another episode (as we refer to them now). We were told like the previous two incidents, Mom collapsed and her vital signs dropped for about a minute and then she miraculously came out of it. She was standing with an aide this time when it happened so there was no hard fall involving any head trauma or possible broken bones. Just as in the past with Shelly, both Mom and the aide melted to the floor. The aide held Mom and repeated to her, "come back Momma Jean, come back. Don't leave Shelly and Whitney now, come back." By the time the ambulance arrived, Mom's vital signs were stable, although her blood pressure was low, (unlike the last time when her BP was high) but she was conscious enough to wave and say good bye to everyone as the attendants took her away on the gurney.

From the hospital, Shelly gave me the report and decided that there was no need for me to drive up there, as they were going to release her within an hour anyway. Not to sound trite, but this being the third episode within a year, even the doctor asked how far did we want to take this. The diagnosis was that she more than likely did have another mini-stroke probably in the same area of the brain as the last two; and since Mom was tired but alert, why run her through a battery of tests? They tested to rule out a heart attack and checked for a UTI. They found evidence of a minor infection, treated her for that and checked her out of the hospital.

I visited the next day and found Mom very tired and somewhat lethargic, but considering what she went through, I was pleased to see her this well. I helped her to the recliner in her room and watched her sleep for a while. I chatted with the nurse on duty and an aide that was present when the episode occurred. The aide told me that when they put Mom to bed last night, she said; "I know something happened, it's the third time."

By the time I visited two days later I was told that they thought she had another episode in her sleep as they found her very bad off that morning. The nurse told me that Mom was hardly coherent and her body was like a rag-doll. Mom was unable to assist the aides in clothing and toileting herself. This time I could tell that the most recent mini-stroke had done some damage. It now took two people to stand her up unlike the past when she would hold onto your hands and help pull herself up to a standing position. She was also very wobbly and unstable while standing, and could hardly take two steps. I also noticed that she clenched her left hand somewhat like how former Senator Bob Dole gripped his pen. I had to physically open her hand and unclench her fingers, as she couldn't understand the verbal instruction to do so. There appeared to be a little drooping around her left eye too. Although these physical changes were quite evident, her personality seemed to be about the same. I hoped that as time went by she would get a little stronger.

I was relieved that a month later, Mom had shown remarkable improvement. During a visit, I noticed that although she couldn't walk as far as before she was back to pulling herself up to a standing position with assistance. She was more attentive and it was easy to make her laugh. Actually, it was a very fun and heart-warming visit.

Another week went by. When I arrived at the facility, she was at the beauty parlor getting her hair done. I sat and watched for a while and noticed that her top denture/partial was not in her mouth. I went back to the unit and asked the nurse if her teeth were in her room. Francy smiled and stated, "We can't win for losing. We finally got them out last night and cleaned and brushed her teeth and now she won't let us put them back in." It was good to see that they were really trying to provide dental hygiene in preparation for the next dentist's visit. I took Mom back to the room and struggled to get them in myself. After a few minutes I had her laughing so hard that her mouth flew open wide and I gently pushed them in half way. Mom got that angry look and pursed her lips, I said, "Mom, you know how to do this. You don't want people seeing you without your teeth do you? Go ahead put them in place. You know how." Well something clicked, because just like that, they were in. She got that annoyed look on her face, and as she was looking me in the eyes I said, "So Mom do you hate me now?" She replied, "How can I hate you? I love you."

The rest of the visit we watched the cooking channel and chatted a bit. I did most of the talking and she did most of the laughing. After a while, I could tell she was getting a little tired so I kissed her on the forehead, told her I loved her and she responded in kind. As I rose up to leave she looked me in the eyes and said, "I want to thank you for everything."

From this point until the holiday season, Mom's condition remained steady. My visits were joyful and less stressful as the care unit really stepped it up. The nurses and aides were doing a spectacular job, and I made sure everyone involved was commended.

Stage 3

It was now February 2011, 4 years since my last journal entry. I don't remember why I stopped; maybe it was because there was a kind-of-calm with this now. During those years, it seemed all of us settled into a routine; we accepted this way of life as our family's "new normal." Unfortunately, Mom slowly deteriorated and became confined to either the wheelchair or the bed during the past three years. With one or two exceptions, the care at the facility was excellent. Although Mom was bed ridden for 3 years, not once did she suffer from bed sores. That's an amazing statement based on the level of care she was receiving. She was hand fed pureed food, hardly opened her eyes and could only whisper one to two words at a time. She still struggled with UTIs, mini-strokes, plus a few new maladies: such as skin cancer, rosacea and Lupus. Her heart was still strong as could be. I visited on Sundays, and Shelly still did her laundry and visited at least three times a week. We both knew these were the final days.

On October 14, 2012, a little past 8:00 p.m. Mom drew her last breath with Shelly and me by her side. Her journey was now over; it was a bitter-sweet good-bye. A few days prior, Mom would not open her mouth to eat. I wondered then, as I often do now, did somewhere in her mind tell her enough is enough, end this ordeal by starving – or because of the advancement of the disease - did she forget how to eat?

-The End-

Afterword: Present Day

Not a day goes by without memories of Mom and Dad. Someone told me that you will always have daily memories of your deceased parents. And that the memories will be positive and heartfelt – he was right. On the other hand, I have moments of guilt, suggesting I could have taken better care of Mom during her journey through dementia.

Also, left in the wake of Mom's passing, is the sad reality that my sister and I are back to where we were 16 years ago. We rarely talk, and have only been together a handful of times in the past 3 years.

I often think, "Is this going to happen to me?" Will my sister or I succumb to the same fate that took our mother? We share 3 of the most important risk factors – age, family history and heredity. Even now, in my late fifty's, I have mental occurrences that mimic some of the early warning signs of dementia.

Sometimes I do not remember the names of people that I have been introduced to recently - recently being within the past couple of minutes, or the past couple of years. I have trouble finding the right words. I often forget simple terms and product names while trying to explain a process or product feature to customers. I seem to be having a harder time with mathematics. Math has never been a strong suite of mine, but lately I have noticed a gradual decline in my ability to do simple "mental" arithmetic. These are all early warning signs, but I am also aware that these periods of what is called "memory lapses" is not a primary memory problem but rather an information retrieval problem. This retrieval problem can be brought on by poor nutrition, stress, medication interactions, lack of exercise, even today's multi-tasking, fast-paced lifestyle.

I will go through the rest of my life hoping that dementia does not find me or my sister. If it finds one of us, I hope it is me. Not because I am the "Big Brother" and I want to protect my little sister – it is more of a selfish reason. I have been the caregiver and do not want to go through that experience again. I can't dwell on it, as that would surely send me into a depressed state of mind and make for a miserable life. I have learned to take everything a day at a time and hope for the best.

As a care giver, one of the many lessons I learned through *Mom's Journey* is that you have to keep your sense of humor and surround yourself with caring, positive, family and friends. If you can't laugh a little through it, it will destroy you too.

Time to Move

More than likely on your loved one's journey through dementia, there will be the time when you are going to need outside help – in-home-care or assisted living/nursing home care. There are three important issues that you will need to address to ensure the route you take will be the best fit for you and your loved one: personality, financial status and medical/health condition.

No matter which route you decide to take – in-home or out-of-home care – your loved one's overall mental and medical health condition will be assessed by the provider's professionals, and possibly a county social worker to assure both parties of a proper fit.

(Because I did not experience in-home care, I will focus mainly on out-of-home care.)

Your loved one's personality is key in helping you decide which option will best fit their declining social skills. In our case with Mom, it was a fairly obvious choice that assisted living/nursing home care would be a better fit than in-home care. Mom was an extrovert, very sociable and loved being with people. (Looking back on *Mom's Journey* there were numerous times that her health declined due to the lack of stimulation and social contact.) On the other hand, if your parent's personality is more introverted, shy or they emphatically wish to stay home with assistance, in-home care might be a better solution.

There are two kinds of facilities: for-profit and not for-profit. In the state of Ohio, for-profit, assisted living facilities do not necessarily have to accept Medicare/Medicaid patients. I have heard of scenarios where rates were raised so dramatically that families were forced to move their loved ones because it became too expensive. This could be very disruptive to the health and well-being of the resident and financially devastating if the family is on a tight budget. Both kinds of facilities are governed under state laws; however, the not-for-profits adhere to the laws more rigidly because of the government funding they are provided. This can be an advantage or disadvantage - as with our situation in *Mom's Journey*, when the state denied coverage for physical therapy. On the positive side, we did not have to worry about unexpected rate increases. We experienced both options, and found the not for-profit to be the better fit for our family financially and emotionally. On the other hand, if your family is well off financially, a for-profit facility may better suit your needs.

Planning and preparing for this move can be a daunting and exhausting task both physically and emotionally, and more so with the nursing home environment. If you have not visited or experienced a nursing home – particularly the memory impaired floor/unit of the facility – be prepared for a major shock.

In most facilities, you will enter and exit the memory-impaired floor/unit through locked doors using a coded key pad. Although this may seem extreme and something you would encounter in a jail setting, the security keeps the residents safely within their unit and prevents them from wandering off. After entering, you will experience a variety of patients in all stages of dementia. There will be some who seem perfectly fine. Some will be bedridden and in wheelchairs. Others will have more obvious medical afflictions such as colostomy bags and compression wraps. There may be patients who have only resided there a short time and have not yet adjusted to their surroundings. These are the residents who will break your heart and cause you to reconsider moving your loved one into the facility.

Upon entering the facility I have had women crying and begging me to take them home. Some asked me if I knew where they lived and would tug on my arm in tears pleading for me to call their husband, daughter or son. I have experienced residents blocking the entrance waiting for their chance to sneak out when the door opens. I've seen elderly men sitting alone weeping and others angry and cursing the staff. On one occasion a gentleman rushed over to me in a panic, begging me to take him to his staff meeting. What I eventually learned that helped me interact with the newer distressed residents was what I touched on in *Mom's Journey* - redirect their attention or go along with them. (With the gentleman and the staff meeting I replied, "Sir, the meeting got pushed back an hour." He then calmly walked away.)

This can be very overwhelming in the beginning, but remember these are the newer residents who have not yet adjusted to their surroundings. I suggest taking a deep breath and look around. You will notice the established residents are just fine. They are relaxed and interacting with one another and with the staff.

On average it takes your loved one around three months to adjust to the new surroundings and staff. For a few days after we moved Mom to a new facility, Shelly and I took turns spending the night with her. We found this to be very helpful with her adapting to the trauma of the move. Some facilities may not recommend spending the night and suggest that it would be best not to visit for a few days. We believe otherwise. You are providing much needed companionship and reassurance that everything is going to be okay. You will also get to experience the level of care provided by the nurses and aides, taste the food, plus, get an overall feel of the daily routine of the facility – which hopefully will give you greater peace of mind.

It is strongly suggested that the family get together and discuss the options available before the time comes for outside long term care. As uncomfortable as this conversation may seem, having an agreed plan-of-attack will pay off in the long run because everyone will be on the same page when the time comes for outside care. This should eliminate any bickering and second guessing between the siblings.

Along with other helpful resource information in the Appendices, you will find the section on "Choosing a Residential Care Facility," provided by the Greater Cincinnati Alzheimer's Association, to be a useful reference. It describes various options and suggests questions to ask in order to match your loved one with their best living arrangement.

Appendices

Montreal Cognitive Assessment Test (MOCA)

MONTREAL COGNITIVE ASSESSMENT (MOCA)
Version 7.3 Alternative Version

NAME :
Education :
Sex :

Date of birth :
DATE :

VISUOSPATIAL / EXECUTIVE

Copy cylinder

Begin
End

Draw CLOCK (Ten past nine)
(3 points)

[ ]   [ ]   [ ]   [ ]
Contour   Numbers   Hands

POINTS

__/5

NAMING

[ ]   [ ]   [ ]

__/3

MEMORY

Read list of words, subject must repeat them. Do 2 trials, even if 1st trial is successful. Do a recall after 5 minutes.

	TRAIN	EGG	HAT	CHAIR	BLUE
1st trial					
2nd trial					

No points

ATTENTION

Read list of digits (1 digit / sec.).

Subject has to repeat them in the forward order   [ ] 5 4 1 8 7
Subject has to repeat them in the backward order   [ ] 1 7 4

__/2

Read list of letters. The subject must tap with his hand at each letter A. No points if ≥ 2 errors
[ ] F B A C M N A A J K L B A F A K D E A A A J A M O F A A B

__/1

Serial 7 subtraction starting at 80   [ ] 73   [ ] 66   [ ] 59   [ ] 52   [ ] 45
4 or 5 correct subtractions: **3 pts**, 2 or 3 correct: **2 pts**, 1 correct: **1 pt**, 0 correct: **0 pt**

__/3

LANGUAGE

Repeat : She heard his lawyer was the one to sue after the accident. [ ]
The little girls who were given too much candy got stomach aches. [ ]

__/2

Fluency / Name maximum number of words in one minute that begin with the letter B   [ ]   (N ≥ 11 words)

__/1

ABSTRACTION

Similarity between e.g. banana - orange = fruit   [ ] eye – ear   [ ] trumpet – piano

__/2

DELAYED RECALL

Has to recall words WITH NO CUE

	TRAIN	EGG	HAT	CHAIR	BLUE
	[ ]	[ ]	[ ]	[ ]	[ ]
Category cue					
Multiple choice cue					

Points for UNCUED recall only

__/5

Optional

ORIENTATION

[ ] Date   [ ] Month   [ ] Year   [ ] Day   [ ] Place   [ ] City

/6

Adapted by : Z. Nasreddine MD, N. Phillips PhD, H. Chertkow MD
© Z.Nasreddine MD   www.mocatest.org
Administered by:

Normal ≥ 26 / 30   TOTAL   __/30
Add 1 point if ≤ 12 yr edu.

Takeaways

Here are a few helpful suggestions if you find that you are the caregiver to a loved one suffering dementia:

- Educate yourself through literature you can acquire through on-line services, library and Alzheimer's Association.

- Don't disregard your instincts when you see changes in behavior. Act on them, you may uncover another issue that needs attention.

- You are the only voice your loved one has. You are the advocate when you see that their care is not being attended to properly. Change facilities if you must.

- Get to know other family members that have loved ones in the facility. You can work together and be there for each other. Especially to solve problems.

- Visit facilities unannounced first. If there is an odor about or if a lot of the residents seem abandoned and unkempt – leave.

- Above all, if you have criticized, remember to commend the staff when they get it right.

- Please do not raise your voice and argue with your loved one. This will get you nowhere. Remember they have a devastating disease. They (like you) don't know or understand what is happening either.

• You are going to experience a lot of guilt. Don't let it eat away at you. Remember that you are doing the best you can under extreme emotional stress.

• Most importantly, set aside time for you. Laugh.

Risk Factors

Scientists have identified factors that increase the risk of Alzheimer's. The most important risk factors – age, family history and heredity – can't be changed, but emerging evidence suggests other factors we may be able to influence.

In most individuals, the risk of Alzheimer's increases after the age of 65, then doubling about every 5 years. After age 85 the risk factor climbs to around 50 percent. One of the greatest mysteries of Alzheimer's is why the risk increases so dramatically with age.

Another strong risk factor is family history. Those who have a parent, grand parent or other family member with Alzheimer's/dementia run a greater risk of getting the disease. The risk increases if more than one family member has the illness. When diseases tend to run in families, either heredity (genetics) or environmental factors, or both, may play a role.

Scientist know that genes are involved in Alzheimer's. There are two types of genes that can play a role in affecting whether a person develops a disease – risk genes and deterministic genes. Alzheimer's genes have been found in both categories. Risk genes increase the likelihood of getting a disease but do not guarantee it will happen. Deterministic genes directly cause a disease by guaranteeing that anyone who inherits them will develop the disorder.

Most experts believe the majority of Alzheimer's/dementia disease happen as a result of complex interactions among genes and other risk factors. As stated above – age, family history and heredity are risk factors that can't be changed. Research is beginning to reveal that other risk factors we may be able to change through better lifestyle and wellness choices. Plus, better management of other related health conditions.

Head trauma: Research suggests that there may be a strong link between serious head injuries and future risk of Alzheimer's/dementia, especially when head trauma occurs repeatedly or involves loss of consciousness. Avoiding activities where head trauma may be prevalent, or at least protecting your brain by wearing helmets while participating in sporting activities.

Heart – head connection: Growing evidence links brain health to heart health. The risk of developing Alzheimer's and VCI (vascular dementia) appears to increase by many conditions that damage your heart and/or blood vessels. These include high blood pressure, heart disease, stroke, diabetes and high cholesterol. It is imperative that you work with your doctor to improve your heart health.

General healthy aging: Try to keep your weight within the recommended guidelines suggested by your doctor. Avoid the obvious pitfalls, smoking and excess alcohol consumption. Stay socially connected, and remember to not only exercise your body – exercise your mind. Research suggests that if you "don't use it, you lose it."

Warning Signs

The 10 warning signs of the beginning of dementia/Alzheimer's are:

Memory Loss

Forgetting recently learned information and not remembering it later

Difficulty Performing Familiar Tasks

Balancing the check book, cooking meals

Problems with Language

Trouble finding the right words, forgetting simple words

Disorientation to Time and Place

Getting lost on their own street

Poor or Decreased Judgment

Summer dresses in wintertime, bad money decisions

Problems with Abstract Thinking

Not able to follow simple directions

Misplacing Things

Put things in unusual places. Iron in the refrigerator

Changes in Mood or Behavior

Rapid mood swings, easy to tears

Changes in Personality

Confused, paranoid

Loss of Initiative

Becoming very passive, lies around on the couch, watching too much TV

Alzheimer's Myths

Myth 1: Memory loss is a natural part of aging.

It is common to have occasional memory problems as one ages, such as forgetting the name of a person you've recently met. However, it can be difficult to tell normal memory problems from memory problems that should be cause for concern. If you notice a loved one with memory, thinking, and learning problems that concern you, it is advisable that you contact a physician. Sometimes these problems are caused by medication side effects, vitamin deficiencies, or other conditions that can be reversed with treatment. Or they may be caused by another type of dementia.

Myth 2: Alzheimer's disease is not fatal.

Alzheimer's disease has no survivors. It destroys brain cells that cause memory problems, erratic behavior, and loss of bodily functions. It slowly and painfully takes away a person's identity and communication skills. It robs them the ability to think, talk, walk, and even eat.

Myth 3: Only older people get Alzheimer's.

Alzheimer's can strike people in their 30s, 40s, and 50s. It is called early-onset Alzheimer's. Out of the 5.2 million people living with Alzheimer's in the United States, it is estimated that 200,000 are under the age of 65.

Myth 4: Aluminum products can cause Alzheimer's.

During the 1960s and 1970s aluminum emerged as a possible suspect for causing Alzheimer's disease. The concern was about exposure through everyday use of aluminum pots, pans, soda cans, antacids and antiperspirants. Since then, studies have failed to confirm any data that supports this claim.

Myth 5: Aspartame causes memory loss.

Aspartame is an artificial sweetener marketed under brand names such as NutraSweet® and Equal®. Since the FDA approval of aspartame in 1966, concerns about its health effects have been raised. According to the FDA, as of 2006, the agency has not been presented with any scientific evidence that concludes aspartame poses any danger to most people.

Myth 6: Flu shots increase the risk of getting Alzheimer's.

A theory linking flu shots greatly increasing the risk of getting Alzheimer's was proposed by a U.S. doctor whose license to practice medicine has since been suspended. Actually, several mainstream studies suggest the opposite. One study in 2001, by the Canadian Medical Journal reported that older adults who were vaccinated against influenza, polio, diphtheria or tetanus seemed to have a lower risk of developing Alzheimer's than those not receiving these vaccinations.

Myth 7: Silver dental fillings increase the risk of getting Alzheimer's.

This concern arose due to "silver" fillings made of an amalgam, a mixture of 50 percent mercury, 35 percent silver and 15 percent tin. Mercury is a heavy metal that, in certain forms, is known to be toxic to the brain and other organs. Public health agencies, including the FDA, U.S. Public Health Service and the World Health Organization, endorse the use of amalgam as a safe, strong and inexpensive material for dental restorations.

Myth 8: There are treatments available to stop the progression of Alzheimer's.

At this time, there is no treatment to cure, delay, or stop the progression of Alzheimer's. FDA- approved drugs only temporarily slow the progression of worsening symptoms for about 6 to 12 months, on average. And only for about half of the people that take them.

7 Stages of Alzheimer's Symptoms

Stage 1: No impairment (normal function)

The person does not experience any memory problems. No evidence of dementia symptoms are detected by a doctor.

Stage 2: Very mild cognitive decline

The person may feel they are having memory lapses. Forgetting familiar words or misplacing everyday items. No evidence of dementia symptoms can be detected by friends, family, co-workers or a doctor.

Stage 3: Mild Cognitive decline (early-stage Alzheimer's)

Friends, family and co-workers begin to notice difficulties. During a detailed medical interview, doctors may be able to detect problems with memory and concentration. (Refer to the 10 warning signs)

Stage 4: Moderate cognitive decline (early-stage Alzheimer's)

At this point, a careful medical interview should be able to detect clear-cut symptoms in several areas.

- Forgetting recent events
- Difficulty performing complex tasks, such as planning a dinner for guests
- Difficulty paying bills, managing money, mental arithmetic
- Becoming moody or withdrawn

Stage 5: Moderate/severe cognitive decline (moderate or mid-stage)

Gaps in memory and thinking are noticeable and increasing. Individuals begin to need help with day-to-day activities.

- Unable to recall their address, phone number, or high school or college
- Confused about what day it is or where they are
- Trouble with less challenging mental arithmetic

They may, however, remember significant details about themselves and family members and require no assistance with eating or using the toilet.

Stage 6: Severe cognitive decline (Severe mid-stage)

Memory and thinking continue to worsen, personality changes may take place, and individuals need extensive help with daily activities.

- Lose awareness of their surroundings and recent experiences
- Remember their own name but have difficulty with their personal history
- Tend to wander and get lost
- Need help dressing and distinguishing proper clothing
- Knows familiar and unfamiliar faces, may forget names
- Frequently incontinent
- Experiencing major personality changes, paranoia, compulsive behavior

Stage 7: Very severe cognitive decline (late-stage)

In this final stage of the disease, individuals lose the ability to respond to their environment, carry on a conversation and, eventually, control movement. They may still say words or phrases. They will need help with their daily care: drinking, eating, bathing, and using the bathroom. They may lose the ability to smile, hold their head up and even sit up. Muscles grow rigid, and swallowing is impaired.

The Dementias

Dementia is the term used to describe a number of mental disorders severe enough to interfere with daily life caused by physical changes in the brain. Alzheimer's is the most common, accounting for 60 to 80 percent of the cases. The hallmark abnormalities are the deposits of protein fragmented beta-amyloid (plaques) and twisted strands of protein tau (tangles) as well as evidence of nerve cell damage and death in the brain. Most people get plaques and tangles as they age, Alzheimer's patients seem to get far more. They also seem to develop in a predictable pattern, beginning in areas of the brain associated with memory, before spreading to other regions.

Scientist do not know exactly what part the plaques and tangles play in Alzheimer's disease. Most agree that they play a critical role in blocking communication between the nerve cells and disrupting the process cells need to survive. It is the destruction and death of nerve cells that causes memory failure, personality changes and other symptoms of Alzheimer's disease.

Vascular Cognitive Impairment (Vascular Dementia) is less common as a sole cause of dementia accounting for around 10 percent of cases. VCI happens due to brain injuries such as microscopic bleeding, mini-strokes and blood vessel blockage.

In the beginning stages of VCI usually impaired judgment or ability to make decisions, plan or organize is affected, opposed to memory loss associated with the onset of Alzheimer's. VCI also progresses in a downward stair-step pattern with plateaus occurring after an episode has happened as opposed to the slow gradual downward curve associated with Alzheimer's. In some cases, several types of dementia can be present at the same time – this is called "Mixed Dementia"

People with Dementia with Lewy bodies, or DLB, is the third most common dementia. DLB symptoms are closely associated with Alzheimer's, but in the early stages have sleep disorders and well-formed visual hallucinations and muscle rigidity, or other parkinsonian movement features. Lewy bodies are abnormal aggregations (or clumps) of protein called alpha-synuclein that when develop in the part of the brain called the cortex, dementia can result. Alpha-synuclein also aggregates in the brains of people with Parkinson's disease (Robin Williams), but the pattern is different than that of Lewy bodies. Again, DLB can occur at the same time as Alzheimer's and VCI becoming a Mixed Dementia.

Parkinson's disease/Parkinson's disease dementia, PDD, mimics DLB in the fact that it too has aggregates of the protein alpha-synuclein. The brain changes caused by Parkinson's begin in a region that controls movement. As the Parkinson's brain changes gradually spread, it affects memory, and thinking, thus becoming Parkinson's disease dementia. Another complicating factor is many people with LBD and PDD also have plaques and tangles – one of the hallmark brain changes associated with Alzheimer's.

Creutzfeldt-Jakob disease, CJD, is the most common human form of a group of rare fatal brain disorders that affect people and certain other mammals. Variant CJD ("mad cow disease") occurs in cattle and has been transmitted to people under certain circumstances. CJD is a rapidly fatal disease that impairs memory, coordination and behavior changes.

Huntington's disease is a progressive brain disorder caused by a single defective gene on chromosome 4. The gene defect causes abnormalities in a brain protein that over time worsen and causes symptoms, such as: abnormal involuntary movements, sever decline in thinking and reasoning skills, irritability, depression and other mood changes.

Wernicke-Korsakoff syndrome is a chronic memory disorder caused by severe deficiency in thiamin (vitamin B-1) mostly caused by alcohol abuse. Thiamin helps brain cells produce energy from sugar. When thiamin levels fall too low, brain cells cannot produce enough energy to function properly. This produces severe memory problems while other thinking and social skills seem relatively normal.

Choosing a Residential Care Facility

Getting started

Choosing a residential facility can seem like an overwhelming task. However, knowing what questions to ask and what information you will need can make it more manageable. There are many types of residential care. It's important to find out which type best meets the needs of the person with dementia.

Retirement housing

Retirement housing may be appropriate for individuals living in the early stage of Alzheimer's who are still able to care for themselves independently. This type of senior housing provides limited supervision and may offer opportunities for social activities, transportation and other amenities.

Assisted living (also called board and care, adult living or supported care)

Assisted living bridges the gap between living independently and living in a nursing home. It typically offers a combination of housing, meals, supportive services and health care. Assisted living is not regulated by the federal government and its definitions vary from state to state. Not all assisted living facilities offer services specifically designed for people with dementia, so it is important to inquire.

Nursing homes (also called skilled nursing facility, long-term care facility or custodial care)

Nursing homes provide around-the-clock care and long-term medical treatment. Most nursing homes have services and staff to address issues such as nutrition, care planning, recreation, spirituality and medical care. Nursing homes have different staff-to-resident ratios and their staff members have various levels of experience and training. Nursing homes are usually licensed by the state and regulated by the federal government.

Alzheimer's special care units (SCUs) (also called memory care units)

SCUs are designed to meet the specific needs of individuals with Alzheimer's disease and other dementias. SCUs can take many forms and exist within various types of residential care. Such units most often are cluster settings in which persons with dementia are grouped on a floor or a unit within a larger residential care facility. Some states have legislation requiring nursing homes and assisted living residences to disclose their fees and which specialized services their SCU provides, including a trained staff, specialized activities, ability of staff to care for residents with behavioral needs.

Continuing care retirement communities (CCRC)

CCRCs provide different levels of care (independent, assisted living and nursing home) based on individual needs. A resident is able to move throughout the different levels of care within the community if his or her needs change. Payment for these types of facilities can include an initial entry fee with subsequent monthly fees or payment may be based solely on monthly fees.

Plan to visit several care facilities. Make an appointment for your first visit, but also make one or two unannounced visits. Look around and talk with the staff, as well as residents and their families. Ask questions and make observations. Visit the facilities at different times of the day, including meal times. You may even want to sample the food.

When you visit a care facility, ask to see the latest survey/inspection report, and in some states, the Special Care Unit Disclosure form, all of which facilities are required to provide. The report and the disclosure form can give you a picture of the facility's services. If the facility is a nursing home, you can go to Medicare's

Nursing Home Compare Web page to learn how it compares to the national average at *medicare.gov/NursingHomeCompare.*

Ask the care facility about room availability, cost and participation in Medicare or Medicaid. Consider placing your name on a waiting list even if you are not ready to make a decision. If the facility will be paid for out of pocket, ask what happens if the person with dementia runs out of money. Some facilities will accept Medicaid, others may not. If you anticipate the need for Medicaid either now or in the future, plan to visit with a lawyer that specializes in elder care prior to moving into a facility to be sure a good financial plan is in place.

Questions to ask

When choosing a care facility, there are a number of factors to consider, including the staff, the facility, the programs and the type of treatment provided. Use this list of questions when considering a facility:

Family involvement

- Are families encouraged to participate in care planning?
- How are families informed of changes in resident's condition and care needs?
- Are families encouraged to communicate with staff?

Staffing

- Is medical care provided?
- How often are physicians and nurse practitioners on premises? Is there a registered nurse on site at all times?
- Is personal care and assistance provided?

- Does staff recognize persons with dementia as unique individuals, and is care personalized to meet specific needs, abilities and interests?
- Is staff trained in dementia care? Is it required by the state? How long is the training, and what topics does it cover?
- On average, how long have workers been on staff?
- How does staff handle challenging behaviors?
- What is the ratio of residents to staff?

Programs and services

- Are appropriate services and programming (e.g., small groups, quiet rooms) available, based on specific health and behavioral care needs?
- Do planned activities take place? (Ask to see an activity schedule; note if the activity listed at the time of your visit is occurring.)
- Are activities available on the weekends or during evenings?
- Are activities designed to meet specific needs, interests and abilities?
- Is transportation available for medical appointments and shopping for personal items?
- Are care planning sessions held regularly? Are they held at a convenient time?
- What types of therapies (e.g., physical, occupational, speech, recreational) are offered?
- Is there a dementia-specific (special care) unit?
- Are religious services and celebrations available to residents?

Residents

- Is personal care (e.g., bathing, grooming, toileting) done with respect and dignity?
- Is there flexibility in personal care times based on individual's schedule?

- Are residents comfortable, relaxed and involved in activities?
- Are residents well-groomed, clean and dressed appropriately?
- What is the rate of falls?
- Are residents with psychiatric illness as their primary diagnosis on the same unit as residents with dementia?

Environment

- Is the facility free of unpleasant odors?
- Do indoor spaces allow for freedom of movement and promote independence?
- Are indoor and outdoor areas safe and secure? Is it monitored?
- Is the facility easy to navigate and find your way?
- Is there a designated family visiting area, or a private place to have visitors?
- Are resident rooms clean and spacious?
- Are residents allowed to bring familiar items (e.g., photos, bedding, a chair)?

Meals

- Are there regular meal and snack times?
- Is food appetizing? (Ask to see the weekly menu and come for a meal.)
- Is there flexibility in meal times based on the individual's personal schedule?
- Is the dining environment pleasant and comfortable?
- Are family and friends able to join at mealtime?

- Does staff have a plan for monitoring adequate nutrition?

- Is staff able to provide for any special dietary needs (e.g., low sodium, diabetic)?

- Does staff provide appropriate assistance based on person's abilities (e.g., encouragement during meals or assisted feeding if needed)?

- Are there any environmental distractions during meal time (e.g., noisy TV)?

Policies and procedures

- Are family and friends allowed to participate in care?

- Do the visiting hours work for the family?

- Has the discharge policy been discussed? (Learn about any situation or condition that would lead to a discharge from the facility, such as change in behavior or financial circumstances.)

- Is there continuing care available within the facility as a resident's needs change?

- Is there an "aging in place" policy where residents can remain in the facility, even the same room, throughout the course of the disease?

- Does the facility provide end-of-life care? Is hospice care available if needed?

For more information, visit: *alz.org/care/alzheimers-dementia-residential-facilities.asp*.

Brain Apps

There are hundreds of brain apps these days that not only claim, but guarantee to improve cognitive thinking through minimal daily use. In 2012 a systematic review analyzed 151 computerized training studies published between 1984 and 2011. The study concluded that certain training tasks had a big effect on working memory, processing speed and brain function.

For the most part, brain apps can't make you smarter or happier, but they can help you perform certain tasks better and maybe have more control over your emotional state. These apps are for people who are reasonably healthy and are not designed to replace mental health professionals.

I am not suggesting that playing these apps will ward off or even slow the chances of getting some form of predetermined dementia - studies are mixed at best. While you are not going to notice any drastic changes, it is worth giving them a try. After all, engaging in new and different cognitive demanding tasks is good for the brain.

The following is a list of some of the best brain training apps suggested by CNN.com.

- **Lumosity -** This app is tailored to memory, attention, problem solving and processing speed or flexibility of thinking.
- **CogniFit Brain Fitness -** This app is designed by neuroscientists. Its goal is to improve cognitive abilities in memory and concentration.

- **Personal Zen** - This app is designed to reduce anxiety by training your brain to focus on the positive and not the negative.

- **Brain Trainer Special** - Much like Lumosity, this Android app has you memorizing letter sequences, phone numbers and solving math problems.

- **Brain Fitness Pro** - This app has a series of memory training exercises that increase focus, memory and problem-solving skills.

- **Happify** - This app trains your brain to be happier by helping to conquer negative thoughts and cope with stress.

- **Fit Brains Trainer** - This app has more than 360 unique games and puzzles designed to stretch and improve mental agility.

- **Eidetic** - Eidetic uses a technique called spaced repetition that aids in improving memorization. This app works differently from typical training apps by using terms that have meaning and context.

- **Relief Link** - This award winning app was designed for suicide prevention but can be used as a general mood tracker. It includes coping methods and relaxation exercises along with relaxing music. The map locator pinpoints nearby therapists, support groups and mental health treatment facilities too.

While technology can help sharpen the brain and calm nerves, true mental health is much more holistic.

References and Resources

Alzheimer's Association *(They can refer you to your local Alzheimer's chapter)*

www.alz.org

Alzheimer's Association/Greater Cincinnati Chapter
http://www.alz.org/cincinnati

Alzheimer's Society

www.alzheimers.org.uk

Fish, Sharon, **Alzheimer's: Caring for Your Loved One/Caring for Yourself,** Colorado Springs, CO: Shaw Press, 1990

Santanachote, Perry, **Life by Daily Burn**, 9-9-14, CNN.com

www.ingramcontent.com/pod-product-compliance
Lightning Source LLC
Chambersburg PA
CBHW070747290526
45795CB00002B/502